REIKI HEALING FOR BEGINNERS

Become Your Own Self-Therapist Using the Best Alternative Therapeutic Strategies to Increase your Energy, Happiness and Mindfulness While Relieving Stress and Anxiety

By
Sarah Allen

TABLE OF CONTENTS

INTRODUCTION

Reiki is one of the highest vibration energy ranges amongst all Universal Energy. Like all others, it tends to harmonize with the other ranges, and it being high vibration is very powerful. It is curative and restorative of physical and psychic situations that somehow do not flow. There are energies that surround us and that we call negative because they are more difficult to master. It seems that they dominate us, not leaving us free to be able to discern what we really want, and how we can achieve it.

Reiki energy is in constant motion around us by wrapping us in full and uniting us with all the living beings of our planet along with the entire Universe. But to be able to take advantage of it, you have to be aware of it, receptive and receive it with humility, openness and total acceptance. With it, we can walk towards integration into the Universe, in the Whole, from our human condition.

Reiki is a millennial medical art, rediscovered by Dr. MIKAO USUI, a monk and dean of a small Kyoto University. Its tradition dates from the Sanskrit sutras more than 2500 years old.

REIKI is a Japanese word which means "universal

energy of life." "Rei" means "universal energy of life," and refers to the spirit or soul to the cosmic energy essence that interpenetrates all things and surrounds all places. "Ki" means "a part of rei," which flows through everything that lives, the individual vital energy that surrounds our body, keeping it alive and is present in every living being. When the "ki" energy comes out of a body, that body ceases to have life.

This word, "ki," corresponds with the "Light" for Christians, the "Chi" for the Chinese, the "Prana" for the Hindus, and also to what has been called bio-plasma, bioenergy, or cosmic energy.

Reiki is a generic Japanese word and is used to describe any type of healing work based on the energy of the life force.

Among the benefits it brings, we can find the following:
- Relaxation of body and mind; recognizing the spirit
- Increased vital body energy and creativity
- Unlocks tensions and unleashes emotions
- Regenerates organs and tissue formation
- Balances energies and develops new capabilities
- Acts on the causes of the disease
- Healing of the whole being.

CHAPTER 1

EVERYTHING YOU NEED TO KNOW ABOUT REIKI

It is very important, when deciding on reiki therapy, that we go to a specialist in this field and, if necessary, do not leave the medical treatment we are already following.

Reiki is a traditional Japanese therapy that means " hands-on treatment." This method was first practiced by Mikao Usui in the early 1900s and subsequently developed by his disciple, Churijo Hayashi.

Reiki treatments have a very noticeable and positive effect on the mind, body, and emotions of the patient. Reiki energy moves through the receiver, balancing its chakras, and raising its vibrational frequency.

This energy has its own intelligence and travels to the parts where the patient needs it most.

Reiki benefits

First, Reiki is a compound Sanskrit word that means universal energy (rei) and vital energy (ki). This practice helps the energy to flow through hands, massages or postures applied by the specialized therapist. Thus, the practitioner acts as a channel of universal energy, with the aim of harmonizing the physical, emotional, mental, and spiritual levels of the person.

Thus, reiki can act at the following levels in the body:

- **Physical:** improving injuries and metabolism.
- **Emotional:** relaxing the person and giving emotional balance in cases of depression.
- **Mental:** helping with insomnia and stress.
- **Spiritual:** granting balance, harmony, and inner peace.

This is a therapy that can be used on anyone, from a child to an elderly person, and even with pregnant women. However, it should be taken into account that this therapy is applied in a complementary way, never as a substitute, for conventional medical or psychological diagnoses.

Keep in mind that reiki is related to the theory of the chakras or energy centers of the body. Simply with hands, the therapist can easily know in which energy center the problem is. From there, they can proceed to work by aligning and harmonizing the energy centers, eliminating blockages that impede the flow of vital energy.

What is reiki for?

Chakra is a Sanskrit word that means wheel. The human body has 7 main and secondary chakras.

With the passage of time, it is normal for our bodies to deteriorate. Thus, negative emotions, traumas we have suffered, or bad habits, can end up hindering the circulation of vital energy through these vortexes of vital energy or chakras. This is where Reiki intercedes, promoting again the correct flow of vital energy and helping to improve the state of health.

On the one hand, when our vital energy is strong, it is easy to find ourselves physically, mentally, and spiritually healthy. On the other hand, when our vital energy is clogged, we can easily become unbalanced or sick.

One of the ways in which we can replenish ourselves with vital energy is by using Reiki. Therefore, Reiki is a holistic technique since it harmonizes and unlocks all the planes of the human being: physical, mental, emotional, and spiritual. It does not attack the body in any way or create addiction or side effects. This is because only vital energy is used, which is present in all living beings; no chemicals or foreign elements are used on the body.

In summary, reiki can be used to:

- Release repressed emotions.
- Provide physical vitality.
- Revitalize the organism.
- Increase the effects of medical treatment when used in a complementary way, never replacing it.
- Reduce or eliminate anxiety.
- Help eliminate daily stress.
- Help eliminate migraines, depression, menstrual cramps, constipation.
- Help cleanse the body and mind of all kinds of toxins.
- Help with pregnancy and postpartum.
- Help animals and plants.

It is not necessary to be sick to use reiki. Therefore, it is a practice suitable to provide relaxation in times of stress. With this method, we can help our body to be healthier, calm bad thoughts, and increase feelings of joy.

Reiki in healing crises

A healing crisis is, in a nutshell, a process that is activated in our being. Consequently, through this, our physical body releases toxins that negatively affect our

REIKI HEALING FOR BEGINNERS

organs, and our mental-emotional body releases emotions and generates negative thoughts.

Symptoms We May Experience

Some of the emotional symptoms we can find in healing therapy are:

- Sadness
- Fear
- Hate
- Anxiety

It is also possible that, among the physical symptoms that may occur, we experience:

- Excessive sweating
- Increase in urine
- Vomiting
- Cold or flu
- Headache
- Fever
- Sorrows of the past

Each person responds to the treatment in a different way. Therefore, usually for a healing crisis to appear, a multi-session treatment must be performed.

A Reiki session

The practitioner's hands become hot with the flow of vital energy, especially when placed on a part where there is a blockage. Thus, the practitioner can know where there is a problem.

To begin, during a reiki treatment, the patient lies on his back comfortably. Then, the therapist uses reiki energy to eliminate energy blockages and balance the patient's life force.

Reiki treats the physical, mental, emotional, and spiritual parts of each person, helping to cure the disease at the root. It can also help the patient set aside the limitation of negative thoughts. Do not forget that continued negative thoughts can become blockages. Therefore, this tendency to negativity can impede our progress in life.

Most people experience a feeling of deep relaxation while receiving reiki therapy. Then, once the session is over, they feel calmer, connected to their ground pole, refreshed, and energized.

Finally, a couple of other things you should know about this therapy:

- First, a reiki session can last approximately one hour. During this session, the patient will lie on a stretcher, barefoot, and dressed.
- Second, during the session, the practitioner can use other techniques, such as massage or acupressure, soft music, and aromas such as incense or essences.

Do you dare to try it?

CHAPTER 2

THE UNIVERSE IS ENERGY

The sages and seers of all times and cultures have always known it, and science is taking a little longer to really understand this: everything in the universe is energy—vibration.

Sri Aurobindo, one of the greatest seers of the last century in India, describes the universe as something that is ultimately consciousness. Consciousness is at the same time energy and a force. The higher the divine one's consciousness, the higher the divine of one's own energy body, its own vibration, and the greater its own power to the point of omnipotence. For Aurobindo, a very important part of spiritual development was the mastery of all vibrations on all levels. He perceived the physical plane as the one that resists the divine transformation the most, i.e., possesses the greatest inertia.

Health, illness, positive and negative life experiences, including accidents and strokes of happiness, are nothing more than a reflection of our own energy field. If this energy field is in a vibration of order and harmony, then the outer life must necessarily proceed

14

accordingly. Conversely, disharmony and disorder in one's own energy field also attract corresponding energies from the cosmos and lead to unpleasant experiences. Contrary to the general notion that we are influenced by the external circumstances of life, Sri Aurobindo clearly shows that our lives are determined the other way around, from the inside out. Mastery in one's own energy field then also means the mastery of external events, health and illness, and possibly even the aging process and death. These findings of a great Indian seer are wonderfully explained in the book "Sri Aurobindo or the Adventure of Consciousness" by Satprem, O.W. Barth Verlag.

There are infinite examples of mastery that show us the potential in our human spirit: when the mother, the companion of Sri Aurobindo, once went up to close the windows with him, since the monsoon rain had set in, she had to admit that the peace in his room was so powerful that the storm could not penetrate, even when the window was open.

Sai Baba, a famous Indian saint, is known for the manifestation of objects that he creates by the power of his spirit.

Indian sadhus master the art without losing a drop of blood, not only to guide a small spear through the cheeks, but even to cut off the tongue with a knife and put it back on a few seconds later without blood flow, and without blood, there remains no scar.

The Karmapa, one of the greatest Tibetan masters, is able to give precise information about where he will be found in his next incarnation, in a letter he writes. For example, how his father and his mother will be called in the next incarnation and where they live.

The crowning glory of all these abilities can be found in the highest yoga of Tibetan Buddhism. The consummate masters of the Dzogchen are known to manifest a so-called rainbow body: when they feel that it is time to leave the body, they retreat to a room for 7 days for undisturbed meditation. After 7 days, only the hair and nails remain in the room, and everything else is transformed into the essence of the elements, into rainbow light. There are various reports of this phenomenon, Namkhai Norbu writes about it in his book "The Crystal Path," Diederich's Yellow Series, ISBN: 3-424-00961-X, p. 178.

H.H. the Dalai Lama has confirmed such cases of rainbow bodies several times, among others in "Dzogchen, The Heart Essence of the Great Perfection," H.H. Dalai Lama, 2000, Snow Lion Publ., ISBN: 1-55939-156-1.

REIKI HEALING FOR BEGINNERS

Well, the patient reader will slowly ask himself, what does this have to do with Reiki? And it is true that Reiki is certainly not about extraordinary paranormal phenomena as I have just described them. What I want to show are the limitations and inadequacy of our previous worldview and the unimaginable potential that is actually in our human mind. And thus also, the spiritual potential, which will be developed much more in future generations, in order to help people in their healing process. Reiki is just one way among many that are rapidly spreading in our time, and support the healing processes with the help of energy and light. Our ideas, our rationally oriented world view to date, are often too limited to explain everything we experience. Therefore, for all the down-to-earth discernment, it makes sense to at least assume the possibility that we have so far understood very little of life, and that we must constantly seek a higher perspective in order to understand. We must keep letting go of our limited ideas along these journeys.

A world view that understands evolution, life in the universe, as an interaction of vibrations, as a manifestation of consciousness—this is necessary in order to grasp and understand Reiki in its full potential.

Even though my ability to really comprehend all this is quite low, I would like to try to build on what Albert Einstein also taught with e=mc^2; matter equals compressed energy on a very low vibrational plane, the potential and the re-use of Reiki.

The Science of Biophotons according to Prof. Fritz A. Popp

... is a further step to grasp consciousness in a scientific approach on its way to becoming matter (and thus also health or disease). Popp's realization in simple terms means: the molecules as such are stupid; they do not know what to do; only the biophotons that move between the molecules and the light = vibration = information = consciousness radiate and turn it into a functioning organism. Popp has shown that food emits different levels of light (life energy/life force) depending on whether it is conventional or biologically produced.

But one by one. Leading in the field of so-called biophoton research is Professor Fritz A.Popp, who has empirically demonstrated with the most sensitive methods of measurement that cells emit light, in other words, there is light in all cells of living beings. We as human beings are in some ways light beings. Popp called it biophotons, and photons are light quanta, the smallest physical elements of light, and bio of bios-life as they control the cells. The quality of this light corresponds to the laser light and is, therefore, able to transmit information. So Popp came to the realization that the molecules themselves are, so to speak, stupid, and only the biophotons, which move between the molecules at the speed of light, tell them what to do. The light field, therefore, controls the molecular field. Thus there is a kind of radio communication in this light body, which ultimately controls all processes in the human body. This light is not only to be found within the body but also outside—we radiate light. It would then be easy to link to the theory of morphogenetic fields according to R. Sheldrake fork, which means that we also exchange light, energy, and information with each other as living beings, without us constantly being aware of this.

The experienced and sensitive Reiki channels will probably only be able to smile because, for us, this is a fact of experience that we absorb and release energies and that the quality of these energies influences our whole being. Both in our own (light) body and in the energetic exchange with the entire environment, we become more and more conscious through the Reiki practice, and one can also say more brightly sensitive or clairvoyant.

With our hands, we can perceive not only the

amounts of energy like the instruments in biophoton research but also the quality, the inner harmony of an energy field. The instruments are not able to do this, they can detect particularly strong energy, for example, in the case of cancer, but the unpleasant perception that this is a sick energy field can tell us that the measuring instruments are always limited to the amount of light emitted. However, such measurements could certainly detect the life energy that a food product has, and Popp has noticed large differences in the light quality of food, depending on whether it came from the supermarket or from organic farming.

Research is now being carried out worldwide in the field of biophotons, and science hopes to find a key to many unresolved questions.

In connection with Reiki, biophoton research is interesting in that it has now been scientifically proven that we are light beings and that light food, i.e., the universal life energy of the Reiki, can positively influence, and even nourish us.

The light of the biophotons controls the entire organism of the human body, so one can even say scientifically that we are beings of light. There is a constant exchange of biophotons, light, information, and life energy between the individual and the cosmos.

Does this mean that Reiki could be explained and proven in the scientific field? But I have, at the beginning, already explained in detail that the seers, the saints and wise in perhaps all cultures and times had long recognized our existence as beings of light...

CHAPTER 3

THE HUMAN ENERGY BODY FROM A BUDDHIST POINT OF VIEW

Mikao Usui lived in Japan from 1865 to 1926 and is considered to be the founder of Reiki or, rather, the Usui Teate. He spent most of his life studying Buddhism and taught his students, depending on his ability, a simple lay version of Reiki, or a higher Buddhist or Shinto reiki practice.

A channeled book by Lama Yeshe (Richard Blackwell), which has been published only in English, explains the medicine Dharma Reiki on the basis of Buddhist texts and explanations from (alleged) records of Usui and his disciple, Watanabe.

(Lama Yeshe had promised an independent review of the (alleged) originals of Mikao Usui until the summer of 2002. However, he remained guilty until the end of the year, which led to him becoming implausible in removing various websites from the MDR, and its students unfortunately doubt him and the authenticity of the teachings of the MDR. Regardless of this, the explanations given on the energy body are quite coherent and interesting, Richard Blackwell has spent many years studying Buddhism and spiritual healing.)

All rights to Usui's texts, as depicted in Lama Yeshe's book, are protected by copyright, so, unfortunately, I cannot provide a verbatim, complete translation to the German reader. But in the following, I would like to make an effort to give a clear representation of Usui's text about the essence of the universe as a vibration, in my own words:

The Buddhist declares our true timeless being, which has always been and is perfect, as the presence of the pure, clear light. If we have really realized this, we are enlightened, freed from the painful cycle of death and rebirth. The Christian idea of a soul punished or praised by God does not exist here, but the knowledge of karma, of the self-responsibility of each individual does. This is on the basis of our own self-created obscurities and obstacles, which are based on ominous action, the pure clear (light) being that we actually become ignorant and tainted.

The Buddha taught the existence of three Kayas, three bodies, and three levels of consciousness, the ultimate subtle plane being the Dharmakaya. From the Dharmakaya arises the Samboghakaya, our human energy body. On this energetic plane, infinitely more or less unconscious interaction takes place between the individual and the universe. The physical plane corresponds to the Nirmanakaya, our appearance.

The impurities in our consciousness continuum cause deformation in our energy field. This energy field, in turn, determines the state of our physical body. This view is not only taught by Buddhists but is also widely accepted in the Western world of Lightworkers. The teaching of biophotons is even able to demonstrate this scientifically.

Again, in other words, all that represents our physical body arises from our energy body, which in turn is created by our own, more or less, painful and imperfect consciousness. Usui cites another very interesting legality: the interaction on the energetic level takes place not only between the individual and the cosmos but also between all the embodied and unembodied beings with whom we have a karmic connection. The interpersonal struggle for energy is also well explained in the well-known New Age book "Celestine's Prophecies." Usui extends this to the connections we have to beings that are not currently incarnated in a body.

There are many examples of this in our daily lives that show this legality, that we constantly (more or less consciously) exchange energies with others. The more we are permeable and telepathically receptive, the

24

clearer our perception in this field becomes. Ultimately, it is karmic causes that make other beings to withdraw energy from us or to direct ominous energies at us. According to the text of Usui, this is one of the causes of illness.

Our subtle vibrational body develops negative, unredeemed areas, which in turn manifest themselves in the physical body or on the emotional level. This is what we call illness. Western conventional medicine is capable of having a healing effect on the physical plane. Reiki, on the other hand, has a healing effect on the energy body, which can then also affect the physical body and the psyche.

The Reiki treatment cannot correct the cause in the body of consciousness, i.e., dissolve the citric stains. However, a correction in the subtle energy body also affects our consciousness, allowing our thinking and feeling to orient itself new and more healingly. This is not only pleasant, but some suffering is necessary to purify body and mind, an idea that we find not only in Buddhism but also in Shintoism and Christianity.

Usui had already said it at that time, which is now revealed in the biophoton theory: every being, whether human, animal or plant, has its own vibration, (I had already quoted Sri Aurobindo on the page "What is Reiki?": Vibration =Energy = Power =

Consciousness). Illness means a false, negative vibration in the energy body, which can possibly be dissolved by the pure, clear, positive vibration of Reiki. The healing process, therefore, involves a change in the vibration, the information in the energy body, which is also caused by bach flowers and homeopathy, for example. Provided that karma can be dissolved, and the individual does not block the effect of purification in the energy body (and the necessary new orientation in consciousness), healing is possible. Healing in this context, we must understand as being pure in light (the plane of Dharmakaya) and not just as an absence of inconvenience to the body or the psyche.

Usui had treated a number of war-wounded with Reiki, and the recovery of those who received Reiki in addition to surgical treatment had gone much faster than those who had not received Reiki. Consequently, complete healing is achieved not only through the treatment of the physical plane, but also in the energy body, order must be restored.

Even more healing in the holistic sense is possible if the individual is placed in the position, through initiation in Reiki, to constantly attract healing energies from the cosmos. This means purification and promotion on all levels. That is why Usui not only treated many people who came to him in search of healing with Reiki, but also initiated them in the first degree. The positive effect of such initiation in Reiki is also not limited to the purely physical or emotional level, but a seed is laid for spiritual development and for a balance of all three levels mentioned at the beginning of this chapter—human existence.

I understand this in the sense that the Tibetan Masters and Sri Aurobindo also taught it accordingly in their spiritual practice: we are particularly efficient, skillful and successful when we learn to master things on the pure vibrational level. The thinking, feeling and the physical body follow this. In the course of years of Reiki practice, we become even clearer and more conscious in our perception. In the so-called invisible, the whole world of vibrations must be discovered.

This text by Usui about the world as a world of vibrations explains very well the statement in his Reiki Hikkei with questions and answers from the collection of Ms. Koyama, that we are working with Reiki on a completely different level than conventional medicine and other known forms of therapy. While they treat healing at the level of appearance, Reiki works at the level of Samboghakaya, which is brought, if possible, in harmony with the level of Dharmakaya. If the energy body is in harmony with the universe, the

27

physical and psychic body follows it. All attempts to understand and regulate Reiki from the worldly level do not do Reiki justice and must fail, because Reiki only begins beyond this level. However, we cannot learn to understand this level until we have acquired a clear perception in our own development of consciousness in the realm of Samboghakaya, the pure energy, and its connection with the Dharmakaya, with the completed truth.

Then Reiki becomes not only a technique of relaxation and activation of the self-healing powers but also a spiritual path that leads to the completion of happiness and well-being, to the bliss of Samboghakaya, as Usui also discovered in Reiki, defined in its rules of life.

CHAPTER 4

PRACTICE REIKI DAILY - FOR A LIFETIME

"The (Buddhist) teachings explain to us what must be realized by us, but then we must go on our own journey in order to achieve a personal realization. This journey may lead us through suffering, obstacles, doubts of all kinds, but this will be our best teacher. Through them, we will learn the humility to recognize our limitations, and through them, we will discover the inner power and fearlessness that we need to go beyond our old habits and patterns and surrender to the greater vision of true freedom offered to us by the spiritual teachings." (Rigpa/Sogyal Rinpoche)

Why do we take part in a Reiki seminar, alternative therapies, shamanic journeys, initiations, and Darshans—all the booming esoteric events? What is the real reason for this? We are all looking for happiness, love, sense-finding, the mastery of fate; let's call it the search for the quality of life. Much is touted to be the immediate solution, the only, the best solution of the inner emptiness. And if it doesn't work out right away, then something else is being tried, and again something else, and in the end, where

29

are we? A few nice, some painful, memories, but nothing has really changed.

The consumerism and rapidity of this time are also often found in the Western world in the field of spiritual search, so I write these lines to show which factors are responsible for the success of our search for the quality of life.

In all ways of self-experience, it is the same phases and the same trials and obstacles that we encounter. Whether it is holistic psychotherapy, yoga, Mother Meera or Sai Baba or the practice of Tibetan Buddhism, Zen or Reiki, what do we do after the initial phase of enthusiasm, what happens next?

So easily we allow ourselves to be caught up in all the distractions of everyday life, all the supposed necessities that have to be dealt with first, but when we die, what is left for us? Can we really say that we have used our human potential with all its lightness and divinity? Have we created causes for future happiness and developed our own being towards the light?

So if we assume that human existence acquires meaning and thus quality of life only when we try to recognize our true (inner) being and try to change accordingly, many external things that we have previously considered so important, and that seem to take full care of our daily lives, will become rather inconsequential.

"More, more, more" is the motto of our outer consumer world, which we are often influenced by. In the inner world, it is more about a reduction, where more satisfaction, simplicity, modesty, and clarity would be desirable goals. Or serenity, patience, the ability to be loving, compassion, truthfulness, etc.

If we take a close look at our lives, it runs from the inside out. Everything that we experience and recognize on the outside, that is ourselves, is a mirror. So if I really want to change my quality of life, I have to change something within myself, and that means swimming against the current of habits, becoming less empty, and more relaxed.

Again and again, we look for new suggestions that do not help us, but rather a patient and persistent daily practice will. And I think Reiki makes it so easy for us. Thanks to the initiation once received, this clear light is always at our disposal for a lifetime, we just need to lay our hands on and let Reiki flow.

Reiki is indeed universal as a practice on the way to light because it nourishes and heals (in the sense of being a heil- =whole) the Christians, Mohammedans,

Buddhists, shamans, and even the atheists. Reiki also gives us strength, blessing, and support at all stages of development. The beginner who tries to relax for the first time, as well as the advanced, who has been meditating for 20 years, does 2 hours of Tai Chi every day or whatever. Always. Both experience through Reiki a promotion in the development of their human potential.

And if I only pause once a day for 15 minutes, look inward and relax with Reiki, I will experience blessed support in the search for quality of life due to its positive impact on my life. Reiki makes it so easy for us, we just have to lie down, then lay our hands on ourselves—without otherwise having to practice an intense discipline and abstinence—and so we come back to rest, into our midst, in balance, in relaxation and regeneration.

In order to continue in the phases when, after the initial enthusiasm, our practice is less of a self-sufficient one, I try to use these lines to make clear what it is all about.

Reiki is a path of self-knowledge, self-experience and self-mastery. "In good times as well as in bad times ...", it says so beautifully, and this also applies, of course, to the daily practice on our spiritual path. It is not more, but rather less (ego, selfishness, self-centeredness) that needs to be developed. This cannot be done without resistance, and one could even say that, by means of resistance, I can see whether I am really taking a step further or not. Integration of one's own shadow is sought in psychology, and this means looking at the pages that are unpleasant and uncomfortable. One mask after another wants to be seen through, and I have to clean up patterns again and again until a new persona is formed, more viable, lighter, and more loving than the old one of the past. All that has been suppressed in the past, perhaps even traumatized from being conscious, many illusions about the inside and the outside, want to be experienced again, recognized, and this knowledge integrated.

Reiki is such a great help, and it gives us unconditionally new strength and blessing, support from above. In its perfection, the Reiki force is able to guide us in the wisest way. But my own mind must also be vigilant and open to this leadership, ready to work on myself, to be mindful that every day becomes a day of quality of life. In many, many everyday situations, the blessing of Reiki can unfold. Life runs from the inside out: if I have found peace within, I experience this also in everyday life. In the end, every moment is a divine moment, and every breath is bliss. But first of all, a great deal is already achieved when I experience that Reiki helps me in one or other everyday situation to be more relaxed and loving, more grateful, and with confidence in the good in all beings, and thus to interact with others in a positive and more salutary way. Each impulse has the property of attracting similar energies, and small steps ultimately have a great effect.

Every Buddhist practice attaches great importance to gaining the right motivation and to remind ourselves why, from what insight, we want to make Reiki every day. The Reiki Rules of Life are a good guide to this, and it is important to also deal with where we want to develop. Occasionally we experience such particularly clear and luminous moments, in which there are no doubts, conflicts, or problems at all. These moments must be recorded as orientation. After that, we often sink back into old (painful and self-referential) patterns. But if we work persistently on our own unfolding, the state we once experienced in a particularly luminous moment will one day become our everyday being.

If today I really tried to be peaceful, without worries, grateful, loving, and sincere, it was a day that gave me the quality of life. If, on the other hand, I have lost myself only in external things, I am missing something afterward, and if I continue to do so for a long time, I must finally realize that my life has become only stress and suffering and that I have the chance to master my life.

I would also like to mention one more obstacle here: our expectations. If we have had a pleasantly relaxing and soothing experience with Reiki for a while, we are happy to expect this as a matter of course. Then suddenly the relaxation is absent, some even think that their Reiki no longer works. That is certainly not the case with a correct Reiki initiation, but our expectation blocks the reception of Reiki. So again: let go, let it happen, let yourself be guided, just be a channel.

Reiki is experienced differently every time and my ego cannot take over this therapy in order to bring about certain effects immediately. In the development of a living connection to and communication with Reiki, we find the same laws to which the connection to the wise, the Divine, and the Higher Self, are subject. In order to understand this relationship and to make it blessed, the study of the I Ging and, of course, the encounter with the Holy Mother Meera, H.H. Dalai Lama, and others were a great help to me. The cartouche cards are also a good tool.

We have so many possibilities here in our Western world, and hardly anyone has to put all their life energy into pure survival, as so many beings on this planet are doing. For all the bustle and speed of Western life, Reiki can help us in a very simple way to take a step back, experience and realize the true quality of life. But we must also (really) want it, strive for it persistently and patiently, and orient our lives accordingly. It is beautiful to be able to fall asleep in the evening with a feeling of gratitude in my heart for all the blessings I have received and passed on. This is a good starting point for the (inner) wealth the next day.

I wish you light and blessing in all your ways.

CHAPTER 5

THE PATH TO HAPPINESS AND WELL-BEING

The Reiki Rules of Life are the only documents we know in the handwriting of Mikao Usui, which state that Reiki is the path to happiness and well-being. What does this mean? What does it really mean?

Suzuki-san, one of the students of Usui still alive today, told us that the focus of the Reiki practice in Japan at the time was to train in accordance with the rules of life in its own spirit, day and night. Also, in the Usui Reiki Hikkei, there is a hint, a statement from Usui, about this. He said, "First the mind is healed, then the body follows."

In the following, I will try to explain this in more detail.

Usui taught a path to enlightenment, to perfection in the Spirit. Reiki, which is popularly known in the West, is more dedicated to relaxation and well-being and healing by laying on of hands. Originally, the focus was on the schooling of one's own mind with the aim of finally leaving all suffering behind, and finding lasting happiness and well-being that is independent of the ups and downs of life. Happiness then means that the inner being, the own mind, is always stronger than the outer destiny. Well-being is also a state of being that takes place inside, in one's own heart.

The 2nd and 3rd-degree symbols are the key to perfection. The mental symbol is the root mantra of Amida Buddha (Amithaba), and "Namo Amida Butsu" is the Nembutsu, the mantra by which the blessing of Amida Buddha is invoked. (Amida is the Buddha of boundless light and, according to Mariko Obaasan, who is a personal disciple of Usui, is said to have been the main practice of Usui. In particular, the Buddhism of the Pure Land (Jodo and Jodo Shin) practices in Amida.)

A direct translation of the HSZSN, which is mistakenly called the remote symbol, reads: "the very essence of being is pure mindfulness." This, too, is an indication of the enlightened state of the human spirit, empty and absolutely present. The coming and going of thoughts and feelings is in this state like writing on water, it also immediately dissolves back into the state of pure mindfulness. The energy follows my attention and intention, and imagination alone is enough for the 2nd Reiki degree to be able to send a remote treatment. The HSZSN is not necessary as the key to establishing a remote connection at all. Usui's disciples learned to experience the Ki of unity in this symbol, which, in the state of pure mindfulness, is a level beyond duality on which there is no separation at all, and thus, everything is connected. Therefore, meditation in the HSZSN can be very helpful in experiencing a transcendent level beyond dualistic, value-giving thinking.

The master symbol of Reiki is a reference to the great all-pervading light, to the lightness of our mind, here too an enlightened state is meant, which must be realized. The master symbol is associated with Dainichi Nyorai, with the Buddha Samantabhadra. This is the so-called Urbuddha, which carries in itself all the enlightened qualities of the five Dhyani Buddhas without having specifically trained them.

When we think of the Reiki symbols in this form, they are a key to entering an enlightened state, in order to train our own minds in such a way that we constantly experience happiness and well-being within us and that all the suffering belongs to the past.

In the application, this means that with the Reiki force, we target our own (!) to develop an awareness that all suffering has been overcome forever. And this is, of course, a very different objective and motivation than is usually taught in western Reiki.

It is beautiful if Reiki even helps to relax a little better, to find a little leisure and inner peace. Lying down and enjoying Reiki is so beautiful. But the potential that we receive with the Reiki Initiation goes far beyond that, and perhaps we should take more care of this and also appreciate it.

In this way, Reiki helps us to connect with the inner teacher and to realize love, harmony and healing on all levels in inner and outer life in inpatient and purposeful practice. Then Reiki, as simple as its application is, is a perfect guide to happiness and well-being, as Mikao Usui put it.

Be good to you !

Usui defined Reiki as the path to happiness and well-being. And that's what we all aspire to when we regularly give ourselves Reiki. We want to feel comfortable with ourselves and with what life gives us. And we want to experience happiness, and walk happily through life.

It sounds so simple, yet it's so hard. A universally valid recipe cannot be given for happiness, because everyone is at a different point in their development, one trying to relax for the very first time, and the other meditating for three hours every day for a long time. And yet, in my many years of treatment practice, I was able to identify and accompany certain processes and learning tasks over and over again. Depending on where we are in our own development, being good to ourselves means something completely different.

And so, I would like to share a few observations with you from my work and also from my own learning process.

At the beginning of the path of self-experience, it is fundamentally important for the vast majority to feel themselves again. Life will only be experienced in thought. One's own strategies of justification, doubts, condemnations and even self-destructive ways of thinking determine the whole life. The cause of the problems is seen only in others and not in itself. The experiences of childhood have led many people to a happy and satisfied existence that has come a long way. To be good to yourself then means to reconnect with oneself, to feel the feelings again, to uncover repressed and compensated feelings, to give yourself a space in the relaxation of Reiki, in which all feelings, even the less socially capable, are one. All that has not been healed and deliberately released in the past, much that has been suppressed and held back, must first be made conscious, felt, relived. Layer by layer, until breathing is free again and all muscle parts are relaxed again. Guilt complexes, feelings of inferiority,

41

various fears, these are some obstacles to overcome in order to be able to feel authentic again. I had to lead many people out of impotence into anger and then on into the sovereign mastery of conflict situations. Some (desperation) screams had got stuck in the throat and had to get out. The inner child, the little boy, the little girl, had been lost and had to be found again. Sometimes the pain had been so great that this part had completely moved away from the conscious personality. What needs healing is no longer present in the body or psyche, and must be specifically captured and integrated with a technique of retrieving lost parts of the soul.

The next step is to embrace good and evil with all that is there, lovingly. Only when I have lovingly accepted the shadow does it no longer lead its idiosyncratic existence as a troublemaker, but can be transformed. And then we have to practice positive, life-affirming, constructive patterns. It's easy, then with relapses into old stories, the mental symbol can be good support for us. Be good to you, but it's not that easy. What's really good for me?

"Be good to you" means at this stage of development, to accept yourself as you are, stop making yourself small, as your father or mother did with you. This is quite difficult because we have often adopted such

42

ways of thinking with breast milk. A replacement ceremony for mother and father can make things easier and show new perspectives. So many parent-child relationships have been manipulative, overwhelming and unloving, and abuse is also a common topic. Reiki can support the therapy wonderfully because, at the same time, we receive very positive, loving and peaceful input from working on our shadow.

Trust is a very important point, even in the Reiki rules of life, it says: don't worry! Again and again, mistrust and old fears or doubt, which is a form of hatred, eat up every new positive impulse. Patience, loving patience with oneself is a characteristic that we must develop. In general, we must learn to be a good loving mother to ourselves, a benevolent, but sometimes also the strict father. Integration is the right keyword, not exclusion and self-punishment, but everything that is in me to accept with the help of Reiki and bring it to the right place.

Only when we have resolved the themes with father and mother, anima and animus come to their place and become consciously tangible. If we can love ourselves again, then, and only then, can we approach spiritual development, orient ourselves upwards, receive higher guidance and inspiration, yes, then we occasionally begin to fly. But a path begins with other maxims, with the themes of self-discipline and self-purification. Then it is no longer a question of giving space to all feelings, but of reorienting feelings and thoughts with care and overcoming all self-centeredness. It is the path of self-mastery, the path of WuWei, of non-action. Compassion and selfless devotion to others are then what we have to strive for, and the good heart must be developed, whether it is a Christian, Buddhist or shamanic.

Thus, if one's own being has achieved a certain degree of stability and clarity and integration, if the psyche can constantly give us positive impulses for the mastery of everyday life, then the path of purification and higher development begins. Certainly also in the initial phase, the turn to the divine light can be helpful, so there is no clear dividing line to be drawn. Often, however, we want to be higher, further, more holy than we actually are. This is not helpful, because our shadow catches up with us again. "Be good to you" means being sincere and seeing your own level of development clearly without embellishment. What I get mirrored in the outer life shows me where I stand in my development. Some simply do not want to see or hear this, they remain unreachable, and therefore they make no progress at all in their healing process.

Reiki, when we have learned again to relax, to let ourselves fall, leads us into higher states of consciousness and lets us experience infinite peace, and inner happiness in a form that we have never known before. Most especially, luminous moments reveal to us our true being. And if we remain patient and disciplined in our daily practice, then this particular light experience, which we have had at an inauguration, for example, will be our everyday life after five or ten years. In this phase of development, it is no longer a matter of simply giving space to all the feelings, whatever they may be. On the contrary, it is beyond being in the world, and no longer of the world. The causes of the problems are only searched within one's own and no longer projected onto the outside world. Then it is a matter of seeing through the nullity, transience, and sorrow of all the impulses we have in mind, not to put them on the back of it. We are detached from the collective, which is a very, very lonely phase, and then we go down the path of inner truth. What we want to develop is, at first, still hidden behind the veil, only occasionally visible. Our divine, eternal being is not yet tangible. We must reverently ask for support and guidance so that we can find the right way forward.

This phase also brings many obstacles and resistances, and sometimes it goes back to the trauma of another incarnation in one treatment. The self-will, the desire to determine one's own life, is a major obstacle and requires many years of purification. Psychic abilities that manifest must not lead to an ego trip or too confused states. Again and again, I have to remember: "be good to you" means to develop a good, pure heart for others, nothing else. Then I gradually develop a spirit that is stronger than the ups and downs of external destiny, a spirit that can endure equally unpleasant situations, if not into positive learning experiences and spiritual growth.

And then... one day ... The veil lifts, and we enter into a life in the light and are now permanently connected with the Divine. The spiritual world becomes our home, our food, our whole aspiration. Completion is achieved when every impulse, every thought, every feeling in us is then good, salutary and blessed for all beings, myself included.

CHAPTER 6

THE INAUGURATION IN REIKI

The most important moment in Reiki is the so-called initiation or attunement, which means the opening and activation of the student to the Reiki channel. Only then can Reiki flow out of his hands; only then is it a protected channel that transmits only Reiki and no personal energy. This has great advantages over other forms of energetic healing: without any daily retreats, diets and other disciplines, the Reiki channel is immediately functional; the transmission of Reiki is always healing and blessing, you can do nothing wrong, you cannot overdose or enter inappropriate vibrations. Provided the Reiki initiation was correct, the practitioner is protected from the sick energies of the patients and is strengthened even when giving Reiki.

Thus, at initiation in Reiki, we receive a great blessing, a divine gift with immense healing potential. Initiations exist in many cultures. Generally, these are transfers of consciousness, energy and spiritual blessing from the Master to the disciple. For example, I have also received initiations from H.H. Dalai Lama in high Buddhist deities and their practice.

47

In the following, I would like to explain some things about the inauguration in Reiki because this topic is not always understood and presented correctly. Some Reiki Masters claim: "Only when you have received 4 tunings to the 1st Reiki degree have you received a proper Reiki Initiation." This is complete nonsense and an unsightly way of supposedly securing more market shares. Usui had given the Reiju—that is, his kind of initiation in Reiki—to the student once, but repeated it weekly. In the western Reiki, there are many different initiation rituals. In the Reiki Alliance after Takata/Furumoto, the first degree is tuned four times, and the ritual to Ishikuro and the Tibetan Reiki is tuned once. At Tera Mai there are three attunements, at Karuna, it is one attunement; each ritual is slightly different, but they all work well and give the student a permanent and protected Reiki channel. So it should be: if you are tuned four times in the 1st Grade, you get a Takata/Furumoto-style initiation, no more, as other Reiki shapes and lines transmit more healing power and a higher vibration.

Many different initiation rituals are known in Reiki, for the activation of the Reiki Channel. And they all work wonderfully, they connect the student with Reiki for a lifetime and have many beneficial and healing qualities for the development of one's own potential and for the transfer of the Reiki power to others.

Some rituals are quite simple; others quite extensive and complicated. The Reiki force is anchored by the master in different positions such as crown chakra, palms, heart chakra, feet and others, by intention, by symbol or via the breath in the student. At the end of the ritual, the student has his own direct connection to Reiki, which is energetically independent of the initiating master. Even the Master is only a channel at the inauguration, a helper, and he holds the space for the spiritual world, so to speak. After the initiation, the student is directly connected to the source of the Reiki and can pass on the Reiki power through his hands, through the breath, the eyes and through mental ideas.

A very important difference between the original Japanese Reiju by Mikao Usui and the western Reiki initiations is the following: the Reiju transmits the entire spiritual potential of the teacher with all the psychic abilities so that the student can access the channel, even with targeted exercises. After the western Reiki initiation, the canal is immediately ready and can be applied. The channel is and remains at the level that the master could transmit; it does not become any more or better over the years; only the perception of the student improves with regular practice. Both the Reiju and the various Western Reiki initiation rituals connect the student with Reiki, but each in its own way.

After the inauguration, it is decisive whether the student also practices Reiki—whether he finds a way to integrate his Reiki applications into everyday life. Only with regular use is progress noticeable, a development towards improved well-being. Reiki is not a sect, and it is up to the student to decide how often he practices, when and where he is completely free. Even if a unique initiation in the (Western) 1st, 2nd or 3rd Reiki degree is sufficient to absorb and pass on the healing power of this degree for a lifetime, it is also quite possible to receive multiple initiations to the same degree and to benefit from repetitions of the initiations. The personal development towards the light is promoted with each initiation. As a master, you can also initiate yourself again and again.

Exchange with other lines of tradition can also be a good extension, and the healing power is actually different in the various forms of initiation. I offer a Reiju once a half-year when I don't see the light. And everyone is welcome to repeat an initiation to a re-received Reiki degree on a donation basis.

And something else: is it possible to remove a Reiki initiation? This is a hot topic. Some teachers say a Reiki initiation is forever and can never be deleted again. Others have specialized in removing Reiki initiations, claiming that Reiki is fundamentally bad. And there are even seals with which Reiki masters try to prevent their students from receiving further initiations elsewhere, a dark chapter in Reiki.

Well, with a proper Reiki initiation, there is no reason to remove it, because it always has a positive, healing, and beneficial effect. But unfortunately, in recent years, there have also been other initiations that are not in order. Where the protection against the assumption of the symptoms of the patient does not work, in which one feels crushed afterward, constantly sloppy and tired, gratuitously aggressive, manipulated, or feels alienated, because other beings who are not full of light have crept in. Sometimes even a brief touch through a dark channel is enough for all the light to disappear, all the joy of the spiritual, and it is a difficult test that people then experience. This can be done with false Reiki treatments, but also with healers who work differently than with Reiki. And this is not limited to healers, even from an English media training and spiritualist association, I know this.

But I don't want you to be afraid here. The vast majority of Reiki initiations are good, and heal and strengthen our well-being!!! Occasionally, however, there are false initiations, which can be seen by their effect. And these can also be removed. As a Seichem Master, I have the ability to do this, and I have been able to successfully remove several ominous initiations, not only from the Reiki but also, for example, the "Light of the Akasha Crown." This is not always a harmless matter, but it is vital for the psyche and sometimes the entire existence of the wrongly-initiated.

It should be clear from the foregoing that the initiating Reiki Master bears a great responsibility. If the initiation has been carried out correctly, it is always healing and is a beautiful light work that has already given tens of thousands of people around the globe an infinite amount. But if the initiation has been distorted, the mental health of the student is endangered. The pupil is also called to carefully choose his teacher and his initiation.

A correct Reiki initiation is a great blessing of heaven, and for very, very many people, the first Reiki Initiation is the first step into a new chapter of life with more light, love and meaning in inner as well as in outer life. The initiation is a central element in Reiki and is given in different rituals depending on the line of tradition. The Master bears the responsibility for the quality, but the student is also encouraged to look for a good teacher and better overcome his inertia.

Western Reiki initiations have a different quality than the Japanese original Reiju, as Mikao Usui regularly transmitted to his students almost 100 years ago. The Reiju is rather a transmission to the development of the entire spiritual potential, not only for channeling the Reiki power. Thus, repeated initiations in the same Reiki degree, also from other lines and from other teachers, are quite useful, and even more, a repeated reception of Reiju. Reiki is a path of self-experience and spiritual development, on which an initiation every time means a special blessing and help from above.

A Reiki Initiation is a gift from heaven. May it always have a salutary effect on all beings...

CHAPTER 7

FEELING COMFORTABLE MEANS BEING AT HOME

Feeling really comfortable in our skin, isn't that exactly what we're always looking for? What do we want? To rest in our own way, to be at home, to be at peace with what is and with what is not. To be stronger within than the ups and downs of external fate.

There is outer life with the fields of work and leisure, family, and relationship. And there is the inner life of our feelings, thoughts, consciousness, and psyche. Whether we end up experiencing heaven on earth or hell depends only to a small extent on how our outer life is going, but much more on our inner condition, on the way we know how to deal with the ups and downs of outer life.

That is why I love Buddhism so much, it shows us how we can train our own minds to experience true (inner) happiness and to free ourselves from the shackles of outer life on our own. And in this respect, the message of Mikao Usui's Reiki and the handling of the Reiki rules of life is also to be understood when Usui says: "Reiki is the medicine for all diseases."

We all know this: If we are newly in love, work is good for us, we fly through the day. If, on the other hand, we are in a bad mood, very simple things of everyday life easily bring stress and frustration. This clearly shows us how much we depend on our happiness in our lives and how we deal with the things of everyday life internally. If I am grateful for all the blessings, I live in abundance. If I do not waste my energy on fears, hopes, and worries, the vitality is fully available to me to cope with the tasks. If I am sincere with myself, truthful and not complacent, I can make progress on the spiritual path and from year to year, make more friends with myself, and feel more and more comfortable in my skin. Reiki is a blessing of heaven, a light and an unconditional love that we can receive every day once we receive a Reiki Initiation.

Relaxing in Reiki and enjoying it to the fullest, leads to us being less annoying, less worried, and capable of feeling the love in our hearts. But what if, after some practice, there is no real improvement in the quality of life? Then we must be more skillful and use the blessing of Reiki to train our minds consciously and purposefully.

It is not the external circumstances that are responsible for the fact that I do not have time, or that anger at my neighbor is in my heart, or that the circumstances of life make regular Reiki practice impossible. It is always my own mind, for which I am solely responsible, that is decisive of whether it is a good day or a bad day. If I take the time and use Reiki for my spiritual development, my life will change for the better. I can become more and more calm, peaceful and loving from day to day, and from year to year. And therefore in the course of life, I can learn to be at home in me, to feel really comfortable with myself and in my skin.

First of all, I have to find a distance to create a space in my life for the encounter with myself, my own mind, my innermost thoughts, feelings, and motivations. The decisive factor is the recognition of how important my inner condition is for my happiness in life, so how blessed it is to deal with myself. Then a firm decision must be made to make a daily effort to make one's own mind lighter with the help of Reiki. In this way, I can connect the worldly everyday life directly with the spiritual. The events of everyday life become a mirror of the progress of my spiritual practice.

The more I have realized the meaning of my own mind, my inner condition for experiencing happiness and fulfillment, the more effectively I can work with myself and align myself lovingly towards the Light.

Reiki is the medicine used to cure all diseases, Usui said. But only if we are willing to change our conditioning, our inner attitude. Usui learned that many patients relapsed after some time because they did not want to change. And that's why he gave them the Reiki rules of life.

Depending on how far we get with ourselves or not, we need to seek professional help to get rid of the programming we are at the mercy of. It is not always possible to do this on your own. Others, on the other hand, can use oracles such as the I Ging or Cartouche to learn more about themselves. And if I have defeated the worst troublemakers in me, seen through mother and father issues, then I can continue on my own and be a teacher and good friend to myself.

With the blessed help of the Reiki force, I can then learn to develop a truly good heart and to tame my own mind. More and more, I will feel comfortable in my skin and be at home in myself. Ultimately, this will have a positive impact on my external life, on work and on relationships. Because in reality, life runs from the inside out. Paradise on earth can only be found in one's own heart, or, as H.H. Dalai Lama said: "The mystical land of the Buddhas Shambala is not to be found on a map, but only in one's own spirit."

With this in mind, I wish you a bright development and good guidance on your way home.

The blessing power of the good heart

or: The importance of an altruistic attitude for one's own happiness.

In July 2007, I was lucky enough to participate in the teachings and the Manjushri inauguration of H. H. Dalai Lama in Hamburg. At the end of this event, H. H. asked all participants from teaching professions to include in their function the importance of wisdom and compassion, the importance of an altruistic attitude for their own happiness, and also that of the whole world on their own teaching material.

What does this have to do with Reiki and the path of Reiki, as well as with faith? To what extent are healing and well-being through Reiki possible in both practitioners and patients, without having this wisdom and compassion in their hearts? I would like to look at these questions a little below.

Mikao Usui taught in the introduction to the Reiki Rules of Life: Reiki is the way to happiness and well-being. This is a common paraphrase in the introductions of traditional Buddhist teaching texts for the path of liberation from all suffering, for the

Buddhist path. Should this also have been meant by Usui? I think so. It is now well known that Usui Sensei has been a Buddhist throughout his life and never a Christian, as Mrs. Hawayo Takata had falsely claimed.

But by this, I do not want to make Reiki an exclusively Buddhist practice, but in the sense of Buddhist spiritual training, I want to show a few laws that apply independently of the religion to the individual and to all who have spiritual healing, happiness, and strive for true well-being.

Usui Sensei gave blessed and healing energy transmissions to both students and patients, but always in conjunction with the Reiki rules of life. Spiritual healing without changing consciousness, one's own mind, is impossible! Healing is much more than just relaxation and often involves not only energy work in the human energy field but also a conversation to clarify the cause of suffering in the patient's thinking and feeling.

Spiritual healing is always associated with a change in the nature of the patient. After all these years, I can say from experience: patients who are full of gratitude, kindness of heart and integrity often experience astonishing miracles in the healing treatments, while those who expect much without wanting to recognize and change are unwilling to see the self-responsibility for their lives, that they have created their own (unconsciously) problem, experience only a little relief and relaxation, but rarely a miracle. Thus, even these healing miracles have a system, are subject to legality, and are thus directly connected with the maturity of a soul. Of course, there is light and darkness in each of us, just as there are light and dark phases in life.

The decisive factor in whether blessings and healing are received from above is an openness to the Higher—to the Light.

The Buddhist defines healing much more comprehensively as a way to freedom from all suffering, to lasting happiness and well-being, to become completely independent of the ups and downs of external life. This is then the perfect mastery of fate, which can only take place in one's own mind. The overcoming of all suffering and enlightenment aspired by the Buddhist means a development into myilucity rather than what is often sought in the world of the New Age as so-called self-realization.

Life means learning and growing; our human existence is a learning process and not just consumption. We must explain this carefully to the patient during the treatment if we want to achieve lasting improvement and not just temporary relaxation. Spiritual healing is thus, in addition to pure energy work, always teaching, a show of the need for higher development.

Higher development, healing, and true realization always mean increasing love, compassion, forgiveness and tolerance. The real cause of the disease, as well as for all suffering, is negative mental poisons, and the Buddhists call them suffering emotions: these must be recognized and overcome. Thus, no lasting cure can happen if the patient does not see his own responsibility and is willing to change. Sometimes this change of consciousness happens by itself in relaxation during energetic treatment, and sometimes a conversation is also necessary to show these connections.

Being able to receive spiritual healing also means accepting the existence of something higher, which is rarely the case in our (godless) world. "Please and you will be given," the Bible says, but this request is not so easy. To this end, arrogance must be transformed into humility, the heart must be purified, and self-righteousness and expectations are also counterproductive. The healer is, therefore to a large extent, dependent on the cooperation of the patient and thus always only the companion. The patient (as well as the student) does not have to believe in Reiki in the first place for it to work, but he must be open to something higher that cannot be subject to his selfish will and control. A certain degree of receptivity is necessary. The greater the devotion, the better.

The central point of this form of healing is the good heart: only with an open heart can it be possible to receive help from above, blessing, compassion and wisdom, as H. H. Dalai Lama taught. To understand this is universal and completely independent of religious affiliations, "Temple needs it in people's hearts," he says. The ancient Tibetan master Shantideva, in whose tradition the Dalai Lama stands, taught: "All suffering arises from the fact that I find happiness for myself; all my happiness comes from wishing this for others." When we look at the laws of karma, it is easy to understand this, and this is a purely logical process, not a matter of faith. Real peace, lasting healing and a fulfilled existence we find in altruism, in a wisdom that has overcome self-centeredness and developed true compassion.

And this applies to the one who is spiritually aspiring on the path as well as to the patient who comes to the healer because of physical or psychological problems. Healing takes place according to the plan of the soul and the maturity of the heart. The real cause of all diseases is to be found in consciousness, in negative, painful emotions and thoughts, in attitudes of life that do not fit into the whole. The Buddha has named them exactly as the enemies of happiness: they are desire, hatred and ignorance. Which brings us back to the Reiki rules of life...

In this sense, I wish you a bright development, good food for the heart, and all the healing you desire.

CHAPTER 8

THE TEACHING CONTENT OF REIKI

In traditional Reiki, there is the first, the second, and the third degree, in addition to the teaching master's degree. Unfortunately, I often found that pupils did not meet basic requirements because they had been incompletely trained in their Reiki seminar.

That is why I would like to try to give a list of the teaching material that a certain Reiki degree should contain. This is based on the most famous western transmission lines and, of course, on my own pieces of training in Western Reiki traditions. Whether you need a whole Reiki weekend or just 1 day for the 1st, 2nd or 3rd Reiki degree depends, in my opinion, on the size of the group and the personal preferences. The pure teaching material with the achievement of the learning goal of the respective Reiki degree is in a few hours and does not always require a whole weekend. Of course, it is always nice when there is enough time to experience and internalize the blessing of Reiki. A Reiki seminar in the length of 1-3 hours is always too short, and during this time, the learning goal that the student is able to carry out the applications independently afterward cannot be achieved.

The Reiki seminars only provide the student with theoretical knowledge and practical applications according to the degree. The actual learning only begins after the seminar through one's own practice. We grow into matter piece by piece; it is a learning and growing process on all levels. And it is a process that takes time, years of practice. It is good if the teacher is available after the seminar for further questions and supervision on the path of the student.

The following is a list of the teaching contents of the 3 degrees of Reiki, which I think makes sense:

The 1st Reiki Degree

- A correct and also intense initiation in the healing power into the 1st Reiki degree.
- A correct theoretical understanding of the mode of action of Reiki is fundamentally important: How does Reiki work?
- The Reiki rules of life are an essential part of the tradition of Mikao Usui.
- A little on the history of Reiki.
- A form of whole-body treatment and chakra treatment, as well as chakra balancing, are included. Intuitive treatment is not possible for

every student to practice the same, so I find it helpful for the beginner to learn these basic forms of treatment. Later on, when the clairvoyance develops, you can drop this form again and treat it purely intuitively.

The 2nd Reiki Degree

- A correct and also intense initiation into the 2nd Reiki degree, which is also intense in healing power.
- An explanation of the healing process in the sense of holistic growth, in order to understand the application of the symbols.
- Explanations of the 3 symbols of the 2nd Grade: CKR, SHK, and HSZSN. Application of the symbols in treatments. A symbol is drawn once and the corresponding mantra is recited three times, not the other way round.
- Mental treatment, Usui called it the "healing of habits." Working with the mental symbol is an essential part of the possibilities of the 2nd degree and should really not be missing, as is, unfortunately, the case more often.
- Remote treatment techniques and room cleaning as well as other possibilities of applying the symbols, e.g. to a specific topic.

The 3rd Reiki Degree

- A correct and also intense initiation in the healing power into the 3rd Reiki degree, into the Master symbol.
- Explanation of the DKM in the sense of perfection of the Mind, a guide to spiritual development.
- Psycho-energetic healing.
- Meditation and possibly also energetic exercises.

Dao Reiki - 1st degree

The High Art of Hand Laying

It's been a long time, but I can still remember my very first Reiki seminar and the joy and gratitude in my heart that I associate with it: in 1987, I went from northern Germany to the Austrian Kleinwalsertal for a seminar of the 1st century. I did grades with Ulla Oberkersch, a student of Phyllis Lei Furumoto (Reiki Alliance), and one of the first Reiki masters in Germany. A whole weekend from Friday evening to Sunday noon in a group of a good dozen participants, all but me from the southern German region. The obligatory 400- D-Mark plus accommodation and food was a lot of money for me at that time, but I liked to give them as well as later 1200- D-Mark for the 2nd degree. I liked Ulla immediately and there was a lot of space and time to get to know the others. It was May 1st, there was still snow in the mountains and we could walk nicely. A beautiful group atmosphere had formed a tense expectation of meeting the saint, and everyone felt at home. Of course, I was told Mrs. Takata's fairy tale of the Christian Usui even then. And for hours, we practiced the same hand positions again, and again, all of them could be memorized afterward.

Today I have to smile when I remember the importance attached to these hand positions. Also, a few years ago, I was in Hamburg with the so-called GrandMaster Phyllis Lei Furumoto, who admonished us to do exactly these hand positions every day and nothing else for a lifetime. The actual teaching material of the then 1 Reiki grades could have been taught in a few hours; actually, I learned little for a whole weekend, considering this from today's point of view.

Only many years later, since 1999, new information about the original reiki of Mikao Usui Sensei from Japan came to the West and so much was put into a different light. It turned out: The hand positions come from Dr. Hayashi, Usui has never used them in this shape. And even Hayashi, after a few years of practice, has dropped these positions and worked intuitively.

So the question alike came up for me: How do I teach how to treat in my seminars on the 1st Reiki degree? — I continue to show my students the well-known hand positions, not in the absolutist form of the alliance, but merely as a helpful framework for the beginner, who can also drop this form of treatment as soon as his perception improves and he can handle it intuitively.

A year or two ago, I came across material from the Jin Shin Jyutsu and the Japanese healing currents, special treatments, and positions based on the ancient Asian knowledge of the meridians, which are subtle energy channels in the human body. These positions can be combined very well with Reiki in a simplified form, without intensive years of study.

CHAPTER 9

REIKI IS PEACE AND SILENCE

That still, peaceful life in our world often runs out, and many hardly get ahead. Reiki, of course, hits a very important point in our lives and can satisfy a very significant and often neglected need. It helps us to relieve stress, to find peace, to go inside, and to feel ourselves again instead of just being in thoughts. Reiki is also so simple: easy to learn and easy to practice.

Many people only use Reiki occasionally to do something good for themselves, or because they are less well off. But we can also use Reiki as a source of strength throughout everyday life to consciously develop further and higher, as Mikao Usui had intended with the alignment of the mind according to the rules of life. Reiki, as the way to happiness and well-being, then means to strive daily for the salutary and blessed contents of one's own mind.

All things ultimately exist only in our own minds, no other is to blame for our suffering. The only trigger, the most important factor, lies in ourselves, and how we react to it. How we deal with life, whether we can cling to or let go, whether we are longing for more, or are content and grateful with all that the day gives us: this is what determines our happiness in life. Reiki can show us a lot, help us, and be a source of strength if we consciously analyze our thinking and feeling, and nourish and maintain healing content.

The happiness of life, the fulfillment of our existence, is always our own responsibility: we can strive to become a little more peaceful and loving every day, to remain more relaxed, to keep a smile instead of being grim, hard, or stubborn. No mental state, relationship crisis, unemployment, illness—no situation is permanent. Everything changes, arises and passes again. If we really become aware of this and learn to let go, we can simplify our lives, as well as increase serenity and inner peace.

The moments of silence are so helpful: to pause, to breathe, to perceive the thought or the feeling and let go again, and to let the moments of silence become longer and longer. This silence must be practiced, and it does not come by itself, certainly not in the urban world in which we live today.

At the beginning of the Reiki practice, it makes sense and is very good to take a longer break every day to give yourself Reiki. Afterward, we are always a bit more relaxed and satisfied. Slowly we get out of the hustle and bustle, and get back to ourselves. Some

71

feelings come up, which had been suppressed. So much that has accumulated in the unredeemed, must first be made conscious again. And at this stage, inner resistance sits part of the way, and they are part of it. After a certain period of regular practice, those who stick to it have to carry a less heavy backpack with them and experience everyday life in a more relaxed and fulfilling way.

Once the calm has returned to the interior, collection and mindfulness have been found, and it is time to observe one's mind vigilantly in all everyday situations and consciously strive for a positive change in thinking and feeling. Then, every situation is a chance to implement Reiki. At the very first moment, I can choose not to get angry at all. If I recognize fears, hopes, worries and doubts as enemies of my inner peace, I can immediately make them disappear from my head before they have settled down or even become a habit. Every thought and every feeling, can be consciously perceived and immediately let go of without any identification with it. In this way, one preserves inner freedom, serenity and also sovereignty.

Out of this silence, consciousness is present in everyday life. If something was less salutary in thinking or feeling, you don't have to go down for it, constantly evaluate yourself or even compare yourself with others: you become aware of what was less coherent and simply choose to make it better next time. In this way, one remains in a positive and constructive state of mind. This is the only way to a stable self-esteem that can exist independently of internal and external factors of neurotic appearance.

And so the same world in which ten years earlier we were exposed to constant stress, fears, worries and doubts, now, constant conflicts look much more beautiful. There is the outer world, and there is the inner world. Both are relative and in constant transformation. Whether one perceives life as joy or as a burden depends greatly on the inner attitude. Reiki can serve us throughout our lives as a source of power, as a light and as a blessing, and thus be a great help to increase positive content in thinking and feeling and to reduce the power of ominous patterns in us. Supported by Reiki, every moment in everyday life can be consciously used to increase the light in us, and also in others.

The mental symbol in the 2nd Reiki degree

The name "Mental Symbol" for the SHK already states that we are hereby healing on the mental level. But what exactly does this mean? Originally at Usui Sensei, it was called the "healing of habits." To understand this, I need to take a little while explaining Buddhist knowledge of the nature and functioning of the human spirit:

The pure nature of the human spirit is empty and open like the sky, in a meditative state. Thoughts and emotions pass by like the clouds in the sky, without the sky feeling disturbed. The worldly spirit, on the other hand, is trapped in the clouds, trapped in desires and dislikes, and ignorant of its true origin, the clear sky. So is all habitual thinking and feeling, the mental symbol in the 2nd Reiki degree. Thus all habitual thinking and feeling, all identification, any expectation, fear, or hope are only as real as we ourselves give them power over our minds. And so our thinking, our feeling is nothing but a habit, they do not possess an absolutely objective reality, even if we often act in this way in everyday life, and thus every way of thinking, every conditioning can also be changed. I can be annoyed or patient. I can react indifferently and dismissively or lovingly and compassionately to any human situation. I can be self-righteous and proud, moody and arrogant, or exercise humility in dealing with my neighbor. Especially in everyday dealings with one's own family or partner, little attention is paid to the vulnerability of the other and there is a lack of mutual respect and appreciation. However, it's nothing but habits, conditioning, the pattern in which we involuntarily function in a compulsive manner, and we struggle to be different in intense situations, to think differently, or less emotionally.

And that's where the healing power of the mental symbol comes in. Its power penetrates deep into the subconscious and can initiate changes in the mind from there, which after a while, also take hold in more difficult life situations and are stable. Pure reflection may often lead us to want to change one way of thinking or emotion, but the power of habit keeps us falling back into the old patterns. The mind is quickly distracted on the outside, the mindfulness is lost inwardly, and already we are again entangled in old patterns and endless dilemmas from which we cannot really escape, with distractions, self-justifications, or rationalizations. With the mental symbol, we have a very effective and helpful tool to finally solve old conditionings and establish new healing ones.

But now for practical application: How is the healing power of the SHK used correctly?

Clear, simple, and very insistent is the method from the original Japanese Reiki, as Usui Sensei is said to have taught and practiced it herself. You sit upright and are clear and free from any distractions in the mind. Without this mindfulness and focused attention on this practice of healing habits, however, this technique hardly works, so the ability to keep one's mind focused is a prerequisite. The Hara is the center of our being, from there everything happens. And so one hand lies before the Hara, the other hand on the forehead. The mental symbol is entered in the hand on the forehead, and in this hand, I also enter the idea of the desired redeemed way of thinking and being. If the hand on the forehead is programmed and charged in this way, I then place it on the other hand, on the Hara, and let the energy act from the Hara in my body and on all levels. Here, too, I am free of distraction; quiet and clear.

In western Reiki, other techniques of mental treatment are taught for self-treatment, for the treatment of others as well as for remote treatment. In most cases, the mental symbol and the power symbol are drawn at the top of the head into the crown chakra, the hands are placed, and the name of the recipient is said three times. Then, the affirmation is entered and concentrated on for a short time, after which the hands remain on the head and let the affirmation continue to act.

So far, this is a very simple technique. When entering the affirmation, however, one should observe certain rules, so that it actually arrives at the recipient effectively and salutary. The affirmation must always be formulated exclusively in a positive way and should be clear and concise. But what arrives in the subconscious is also always the whole image, the felt idea that is entered! As we recite the phrase affirmation, the image and feeling must also be purely positive and redeemed, because this works much more than the words we say.

When someone enters: "I am patient and loving in the care of the mother-in-law," but actually feels: "Oh God, the poor, now she also has to look after the mother-in-law," the latter arrives and makes them depressed rather than happy. We must, therefore, take great care that the emotional energy and the presented image are also redeemed during the input, and are purely positive. The emotional energy affects the receiver even more than the energy imaginable. When we know this and use it accordingly, the mental treatment is very powerful and can convert many old habits into new redeemed ones. So a sentence should not only be said but there should be an intensely felt (!) presentation in conjunction with the sentence. Then, such a mental treatment is very effective and beneficial.

In most cases, a whole series of mental treatments with the same affirmation is recommended on consecutive days, preferably in the morning, at noon and in the evening, so that even deep-seated habits can be changed. I always recommend a book about affirmations by Louise L. Hay: "Heal Your Body." In this small booklet, body areas and illnesses are psychosomatically assigned to the wrong unredeemed ways of thinking, and suggestions are given for corresponding positive affirmations. The assignment of the individual vertebrae to body zones and ways of thinking is also helpful and revealing for the professional practitioner.

After a mental treatment, it makes sense to keep silent about it, so as not to draw disturbing thoughts of others to this healing process. As is so often the case with spiritual exercises, all beginnings are slightly endangered by external influences of the doubt of third parties. The thoughts of others can have a disturbing effect on one's own development. This is the reason for secrecy, that one keeps silent about things such as a mental symbol, even certain Buddhist teachings and certainly initiation experiences, and does not talk about it with those who are far-left.

After years of practice, faith in the light is confirmed many times by experience, a powerful connection is established on the inner plane to the spiritual world, and then we are also so consolidated that thoughts of others can no longer make us waver. In this sense: May your heart connection to the light strengthen and intensify a little more every day, and may all the healing that you want, happen, according to the plan of the soul.

CHAPTER 10

PRACTICE DAILY FOR A BETTER WORLD

H. H. Dalai Lama is an embodiment of Avalokiteshvara, the Buddha of infinite, perfect compassion. The Dalai Lama is tireless in his quest to help all beings in the best possible way, out of pure, selfless compassion with all suffering beings. The radiance of such a consummate saint is probably not unaffected.

Towards the end of the event in Nottingham in May 2008, the Dalai Lama was asked the following question from the audience: "H. H. was so kind to us, how can we do something for Him?" And his answer was direct and clear: "Practice sincerity! Become more harmonious and create a better world."

This shows parallels to the Reiki rules of life and can also be applied to our daily Reiki practice. This is what all spiritual traditions are all about. This is the essence of the search for the Higher and for a sense of life: tame your own mind, develop a good heart, and thus make the world a little more loving.

Developing the quality of heart is what it really is all about. And that is perhaps the only thing that can actually make our world better and more beautiful, both inside and out. In the New Age, a person who can almost fly has incredible clairvoyance abilities etc., and a higher species with advanced magical and psychic traits were sometimes predicted for 2012. It is often overlooked that these properties are only a side effect, and if the self identifies with them, they are even an obstacle on the path of higher development, because the essence has always been the same since the beginning of the day: the quality of the heart develops through Self-mastery, devotion and purification. The result is completely unspectacular and reveals itself precisely by its simplicity.

What does this mean? It means to regard the others more important than learning humility, to reduce one's attachment and defense, and to be more compassionate and loving in dealing with all, no matter how they behave towards us. The Holy Mother, Meera, says, "Become a little more loving and peaceful every day."

But how can we implement this in everyday life? We have to motivate ourselves first: Why did I start Reiki? What am I looking for? What happiness do I want to experience in life? What really matters in my life? And then it quickly becomes clear that, on the one hand, we have ups and downs in external life that can only be controlled to a limited extent, but ultimately the internal constitution decides whether or not we are satisfied and happy with what is and what is not. In this way, we realize how helpful and significant daily Reiki practice is.

Of course, it is also perfectly okay if you only give yourself Reiki occasionally, when something is hurting, you feel miserable or just want to relax a little bit. But a development towards heart quality, and increased well-being and happiness in life requires more effort and as regular reiki as possible, especially on days we don't really like and prefer distraction.

The inauguration in Reiki is a great gift from heaven, it is made so easy for us: to lie down, lay hands, relax and feel good, to just let it happen, and let go. And afterwards, we are in a more loving and peaceful constitution. This is done on its own. But of course, we can also do more and always align ourselves with the rules of life in everyday life, using Reiki as a source of strength for our own process of higher development. All beginnings are difficult, but if I have consciously exercised patience in place of anger a few times, this too becomes a habit. When I realize what a beautiful divine blessing I have received through the Reiki Initiation, I remain in humility and gratitude, and so more and more blessings can happen. And in times when I struggle, I recognize the value of sincerity towards myself. Only in this way, I can continue along the path.

Reiki helps us to nourish so much inner peace and a warm, kind heart so that we can feel love and compassion in our hearts, and this also has a beneficial effect in all our encounters. This, in turn, also comes back and strengthens us. After 10 years, our life looks very different, both inside and outside the light of the soul begins to shine. H. H. Dalai Lama would also enjoy this ...

The hand positions in the Reiki

Since 1999 we have learned that Reiki still exists in Japan and that Mikao Usui has encouraged his students from the very beginning to be intuitive in the treatment and either let their hands be completely guided by Reiki or to use the hands to identify energetic disturbances in the human energy field and then treat them in a targeted manner. Hayashi, as a former doctor, first developed position sequences for certain diseases, but dropped them in later years and instead worked only purely intuitively. Ms. Takata met hand positions at her Reiki treatments in Tokyo, brought them to the West, and either herself or her granddaughter Furumoto then declared this sequence of treatments absolute.

We know more about Suzuki San, who has been with Usui for 12 years, as opposed to Hayashi, who has only witnessed the last 9 months of Usui: Usui has worked intuitively, much more purely mentally, so without direct contact. From the very beginning, he taught his students to work intuitively, to learn to distinguish energy fields in the body. And this ability was also particularly supported and promoted by the regular Reijus, the original form of initiation that Usui has repeatedly given to his disciples, and which is very different from the western form of initiation in Reiki.

A special form of treatment, but rather unsuitable for the beginner, was actually used by Usui Sensei, according to Suzuki San. I find this magical, and it is incredibly effective: without touching the body at all, all meridians, all zones, all organs, all systems, all levels of man are treated via only 5 imagined head positions. Combined with the blessing of the healing Buddha Binzuru, there are 5 mudras that are imagined at the head of the recipient and treat specifically all 12 meridians in the body. If my information about Reiki in Japan is correct, in Usui's time, this is the only original Reiki treatment form, apart from the purely intuitive treatment. It is much more difficult to apply than western whole body treatment, but it also goes much deeper and is more comprehensive. Their healing effect amazes me again and again. And so you also train the ability to see the meridians directly in the body and then place energies in disturbed areas of a meridian. However, this type of treatment requires mental abilities in order to be effective accordingly.

For a professional treatment, I discovered another treasure a few years ago: treatment points on the meridians, as they are applied in Japanese healing streams and in Jin Shin Jyutsu. This is the main subject of the seminary Dao Reiki 1. Here, as in an apprenticeship as a physiotherapist, the student must be able to learn a lot about the respective position and also in treatment, which of the 18 positions is the one that the client needs at the moment. Then it can be worked very effectively, and one or two of these hand positions achieve more than several whole-body treatments according to the classic traditional Western Reiki system.

CHAPTER 11

REIKI IN THE PRESENT DAY, REIKI FOR THE EXHAUSTED SELF

The achievements of modern civilization allow us to live more and more in a man-made artificial world, in a world away from nature, away from natural rhythms and far from silence and pause. Has man really improved his world with it? Environmental protection has found its place and is trying to limit the damage caused by the exploitation of the planet. But what protects people's minds and psyches? Modern medicine and psychology speak of new diseases such as ADHD (attention deficit syndrome), anxiety neurosis (pain of social isolation) and CFS (chronic fatigue syndrome), and now also of the exhausted self. The exhausted self—a symptom of our modern meritocracy—and how Reiki can be helpful and healing should be the subject of this book.

The human psyche has also long been under pressure to perform in the economy, which is constantly geared towards growth. The classic definition of economics is a system for meeting human needs. This has become completely self-sufficient and a system of creating more and more needs that never end. But should we not then be allowed to ask the question, to what extent this system actually increases human happiness or even destroys it? Bhutan is the only state on the planet that has anchored the pursuit of inner happiness at the forefront of its legislation and political leadership. But this is not to become a political text, only the background of the social system in which we spend our daily lives should be pointed out for a short time so that we can see to what extent we ourselves are manipulated by it or not. The external life of increasing productivity has also had an impact on the inner level of man, and stress is part of everyday life; nature is a luxury.

Outer inspiration is also reflected on the inner plane: an always strenuous attitude in life, one's own self must always get better, and the persona constantly optimized. This restless optimization of the self, whether conscious or unconscious, leads to the fact that hardly anyone can love and accept themselves as they are. But also, the handling of oneself is performance-oriented up to the grotesque spectacle of his own body to further and further optimize the gender marketplace in order to have better chances of winning. So many people are becoming more and more estranged from themselves. They are only in their heads and without connection to the heart and their belly. Once they pause the constant distraction and pressure to perform, they find only emptiness, futility, and have no connection to themselves, only to the optimization goals of their self. Inner satisfaction, which accepts everything lovingly and gratefully as it is, seems to exist only on another planet.

It is not surprising that the demand for therapy in both classical and alternative forms has increased very strongly at the moment. Especially the interest in all kinds of life support, in order to find a way of self-therapy, and to reconnect with the inner being and a sense of life within itself. Always being at work, won't work in the long run. But to pause and simply enjoy the moment in the here and now as it is, is very difficult.

The strenuous attitude has become a powerful habit; the miraculous and fulfilling experience that was lingering in the unity of giving has come a long way. Instead, most feel overwhelmed, not good enough for this world, they orient themselves to external things and have lost touch with their own inner beings. Heart and stomach have to function according to the ideas and expectations of rational thinking, and their messages are ignored (if there is a pain signal, just take a tablet and carry on). On the other hand, if one senses inwardly and gives space and attention to the inner conflicts and alternating impulses, a solution can be found even without the control of thought. As the saying goes: Only with the heart one sees well. This is also to be applied to the handling of oneself! But if everything is conducted only from the head and is always tensely subordinated to the striving for optimization, the inner conflicts manifest themselves as illness and pain, and our modern society also has its typical modern diseases such as ADHD, Anxiety neurosis, cancer and allergies. The new psychological concept of the exhausted self is a sign of the times, a signal for rethinking: this is simply no longer the case, the vitality is exhausted, nothing is possible anymore. How long must one have disregarded the messages of the body in order to get to this point?

Sometimes we feel that balancing and switching off are important, that we have to relax again and leave the pressure of performance and optimization behind. Regenerating and letting go at all levels is possible, to the point of the desire for nothing more, which alone can really give us peace. Reiki can be very helpful and healing for everyone. You can go to a practitioner and also get Reiki treatments, attend a Reiki seminar and from then on, give yourself reiki every day. Reiki is easy to learn and practice, and there are no exceptions at all; anyone can do this. Reiki helps us to go inside again, to feel ourselves again instead of just thinking. Reiki is regenerating, brings back calm and strengthens all levels and systems of man. And there is nothing wrong: For Reiki directs, guides, leads and lets everything happen, so one does not work with one's own will or energy but is a channel for a pure divine light that always works salutary on all levels.

Many people are looking for something that will help them to find themselves again, and Reiki is ideal because it can be learned in a few hours and enjoyed without any special effort during treatment or self-treatment. Reiki takes over the work, so to speak, we just have to let it happen. The universal life energy that we receive in a Reiki treatment strengthens us on the energetic level and supports any form of development of our own potential. Whether you are spiritually oriented or not, old or young, sick or healthy, Reiki can give something to everyone in his or her own individual way through life. With Reiki, we can easily take a break to regenerate and find ourselves again. Finally, we can switch off again. Even the exhausted self can lie down to Reiki and treat itself, thereby regaining strength and meaning. However, a good practitioner can also support this process of healing the soul particularly well by seeing exactly where the person is standing, making him aware of this, and then pointing out targeted solutions.

Sometimes there is not so much that needs to be changed in one's own life in order to be able to experience peace and contentment again. Only a little space is needed for Reiki, for pause, and to find one. The exhausted self needs food from within, a space without incitement, where self-love and value-free acceptance of all that one is will be experienced as a counterpoint to all the demands that outer life places on one. In this way, the exhausted self can find its way home, and relive being at home. Reiki is a very simple and perfect way to create this space in your everyday life and to come back home.

Sometimes, the beginning is not so easy, because, like addicts, people are directed outward and programmed for consumption and distraction. Often it takes a life crisis to wake up and ask yourself: Isn't there anything else that can make me happy and satisfied? A distraction-free silence and a direct encounter with oneself, can hardly be endured and inside feels empty and dead. Some have completely lost touch with themselves in their wholeness. But even at this point, Reiki makes it very easy for us to regain access to ourselves. Reiki is then an inexhaustible source of power, which builds us up every day and supports us on our way. It gives us peace and relaxation, light and blessings.

CHAPTER 12

WIRELESSLY HAPPY? REIKI SHOWS US HOW

Some Reiki students were rather skeptical at the beginning of their first Reiki seminar, but in the end, everyone had an inner experience that Reiki is doing well. In any case, I know only one instance from my almost 15 years with infinite reiki initiations, where the doubtful spirit was so overpowering that nothing had been experienced except for one's own neurosis.

However, the differences in how Reiki works and how it is experienced are great, and one can relax very well and drop very quickly the other struggles experienced with it at first. Even with the same person, Reiki is experienced differently and anew every time. So we need patience, and then it becomes easier and the condition in everyday life becomes more relaxed and lighter. If the Reiki student finds a way to integrate Reiki into his everyday life and regularly practice Reiki, only then will a positive change in the inner and outer life take place. The eyes begin to glow and get depth—the depth of the soul.

Those who practice Reiki seriously will make progress year after year, and it is a growth process in which all levels of the human being participate. And occasionally, there are particularly deep and dissolved states in which one never wants to reappear. This is not possible, but it is possible to become aware of the quality of this state and to aspire to it in the further life as the truth, as the light, as the essence of being, or as Usui defined it in the introduction to the Reiki rules of life. : As the path to happiness and well-being, which is a classic description of the Buddhist path, liberation from all sufferings and the realization of the spirit of enlightenment.

Many Reikians have experienced such a little satori before, but the meaning has not become clear to them at that moment. In deep relaxation, all worries fall, all fears disappear, there is nothing to be annoyed about, love in the heart is there for all and also gratitude. This IS the truth: no more ego and no more will or pushing away; everything is okay as it is. The distinction between I and You also dissolves, and we experience unity.

Many experienced such conditions in the Reiki, and yet they went down again as soon as the treatment was over, and discursive thinking had regained the upper hand. It's a pity because we could learn so much from it. It is possible to be unconditionally happy, to be at home within so that one is no longer looking for something outside. It is a state of desirelessness, an experience of undesired happiness.

In Buddhist doctrine, Dukha is spoken of, which means as much as not fulfilled—unsatisfied. All-consuming thinking, and all desires create tension. And so, in the end, we live our whole lives in a state of Dukha, of non-fulfillment. Everything you desire creates tension and restlessness. In the deep relaxation that Reiki sometimes gives us, we come into this state of desirelessness, the outer life is still the same, and yet it can no longer disturb our inner peace.

You experience such a feeling of deep peace in the Reiki, everything dissolves and falls away from you, why then do you start to put so much stress on yourself afterward? Reiki shows the way to happiness, to inner happiness in the heart. There is nothing more to be desired, hoped for, or feared. There is only the pure being, the being in the here and now, in unity.

Any deep relaxation in Reiki can show us that there is another way to happiness and well-being, to happiness without desire. Well, if one is made aware of this again and again and aligns one's own mind according to it, then year after year, even higher enlightened experiences of being can arise, in perfection that one cannot yet imagine. It is always up to ourselves, whether we aspire to this inner happiness in our hearts or the world of external desires. Reiki shows us the way inward.

Reiki - the path to happiness and well-being

Reiki treatment is soothing and very pleasantly relaxing, easy to use without being able to do anything wrong, and without having to train for years. And so it is very helpful even in today's hectic times to be able to reduce stress in this way and to come back a little to rest. Traditionally, the 1st Reiki seminar teaches different ways of laying on hands in order to be able to treat oneself and others with Reiki. In addition, the Reiki rules of life are always an essential part of the daily Reiki practice.

However, the potential of the Reiki is far from being reached, the introduction to the Reiki Rules of Life states: Reiki is the "path to happiness and well-being." It is probably no coincidence that this very formulation was chosen by the founder Mikao Usui. The "path to happiness and well-being" is a classic description of the Buddhist path, the way to liberation from all sufferings and the pursuit of enlightenment.

And so, for the practice of Reiki, we can also use some very basic rules of Buddhist lifestyle and thinking, without having to change religion and take refuge in Buddhism. The Buddha's teaching shows us the laws according to which true well-being and happiness of life are to be attained, according to which our being, which is primarily spirit, functions. The better we understand how our minds work and thus shape our destiny, the better we can consciously develop with Reiki.

The pursuit of happiness is universal; all living beings have this in common and desire this. For the intelligent Homo Sapiens, lasting and stable happiness is to be found less in the outside than in one's own mind, as the Reiki rules of life point out to us.

Reiki, as our universal source of power, can be used even better in everyday life by realizing how our minds work and then training our own minds to get used to positive attitudes that are helpful and healing.

Only when one becomes aware of the phenomena working in one's own psyche can one also transform them and take a lighter and more loving path. The inner troublemakers, the emotional and mental constraints, can be gradually purified by loving and constructive dealing with one's own being until they lose their power over you.

Our self-image is usually a neurotic element, which always has one's own self first in its attention, and either makes itself larger and more important out of this self-relationship, combined with an unrealistic and unteachable self-righteousness, or making itself smaller and less inferior, which can be increased to self-pity and the play of the poor self. Both neurotic components of our minds must first be recognized and then overcome in a clever way. But how???

Reiki teaches us to let go: If I do not follow these thought processes of self-centeredness further, but let them move on relaxed again, then calm and associated clarity will arise. Then, I can experience myself as big and small, without my self-esteem changing. Thereafter all the attention is no longer used to make myself bigger or smaller, but I can begin to constructively establish a connection with myself, at the end of which I no longer take myself so seriously but have realized that my own Well-being depends on how far I love others in my heart and am more interested in their happiness than my own.

How much stress is there every day around this self-image? How much am I trapped in pride or in compensating or rationalizing thought patterns, and can lose my composure so quickly? How many times has the self-image changed, everything seemed great when it was a good day, or horrible when my hypocrisy had suffered? So much revolves only around one's own self-image, which ultimately turns out to be pure conceit, but which is often difficult to see through.

All these projections and fixations, the Buddha calls spiritual poisons, that come from the patterns of fear and hope, from the will to have or the defenses. I can be conscious of every single reaction in my being and try to see through it, so I modify my attention inward rather than outwardly: How much true happiness and well-being does this habitual reaction really give me?

It is very important in this self-experience that we treat ourselves lovingly, that we learn to be a good "Reiki" friend to ourselves: "Okay, that was not good, tomorrow we will do better." And then let go again. So I stay on a constructive level with myself. I find a wise and loving way of dealing with the self, and that feels much more beautiful than constantly getting bigger or smaller, or even going into guilt complexes or devastating thoughts out of self-rejection.

Inward attention makes us realize how quickly we want to reach for something that promises amenity or to fend off something that goes against the grain of self-centeredness. This is how we live in the constant change of fear and hope. The path of Reiki, on the other hand, can show us how beautiful it is to be loving, grateful and serene simply by letting things be as they are. This is great art if we have fully internalized this, we are enlightened and free from all sufferings.

The more one deals with the importance of the Reiki rules of life for the daily practice of Reiki, the more it becomes clear that this is a long way, that it is spiritual development, and that this, in turn, means recognizing the tyranny of the ego in the first place, and ultimately defeat. The Spirit is constantly concerned with fear and hope, with desire and defenses and is extremely tricky in this endeavor. This requires sincerity towards oneself—the fourth of the rules of life. "Don't worry today" means something else: to actually use your mind skillfully and not to constantly worry about superfluous and stressful thoughts.

Reiki helps us every day to come into serenity, to look carefully into the here and now, mindful of the inward and is an inexhaustible source of strength on this journey. Using Reiki gives us a blessing that simplifies and makes life more beautiful, lighter, and more loving.

May all the healing you want, happen according to the plan of the soul.

CHAPTER 13

THE REIKI-GRADE

Defining the term "Reiki" clearly and universally, and in doing so thinking more than receiving and transmitting light, is quite difficult in all the different forms that are taught and practiced under the name Reiki. And the "scholars are also at odds with each other" on a definition of the term Usui Reiki that is valid for all. Usui Reiki is also available in many variants, in Western and Japanese traditions.

One of the characteristics of all traditions of Reiki is that it is taught in three successive degrees—Reiki 1, Reiki 2, and Reiki 3. Also, in the writings of Mikao Usui, the founder of Reiki Ryoho, the Reiki healing method, there are three degrees, three levels in which he taught his disciples, namely, shodes, okudes and shinpads. In terms of content, however, these deviate from the degrees that have spread widely in the Western world known as Reiki 1, 2 and 3.

The first Reiki degree (in Western traditions) allows the introduction to reiki practice. In addition to a theoretical understanding of how it works, intention, and history teaches the student the practical application by placing his hands on both his own body and another person's. A one- to one-and-a-half hour full-body treatment with certain hand positions and a short chakra treatment are part of a Reiki-1 seminar. So are the ideals, the Reiki rules of life, the prayer that Mikao Usui and his students recited to common practice.

After the seminar, the actual practice begins for the student, because only if Reiki is applied in a reasonably regular form in everyday life, can its blessing and healing power have an effect on personal development and general well-being. The practice of hand laying after the inauguration to the Reiki canal means not only an increased opening of the hand chakras from which Reiki flows out but, as is the case with all the other chakras of the human energy body, the hands will also be used in the course of the time to become a trained perceptual organ for energetic vibrations.

If, after a certain period of Reiki practice, the whole being has opened up to the light of Reiki, there is an interest in further applications and a certain sensitivity to the flow of energy has been developed, the student is ready for the second Reiki degree. This may take half a year or a whole year, but it varies quite differently individually.

In the second Reiki degree, there are symbols that make specific energies available. Their applications are taught and three symbols are common, namely, a force symbol, a mental symbol, and a so-called remote symbol. With the help of these symbols, the Reiki 2 student can give more targeted, comprehensive, effective, and much more powerful treatments, as well as energetic room cleaning, remote treatments, mental treatments far beyond the reach of his own hands and much more. The power symbol alone reinforces its Reiki many times compared to the first degree.

Other symbols for grounding, karmic healing, inner peace, the purification of psychic energy and angelic work, and a symbol for back treatment are added to the 3 traditional Reiki symbols. These are from Tera Mai and Karuna Reiki, respectively.

Even after the Reiki 2 seminar, one's own practice and experience are very important, because it is only in the course of time that we grow into this world of the so-called invisible and are able to develop a clear perception in the realm of energies and vibrations. This goes hand in hand with one's own spiritual and emotional development and is a process that takes time. It is an inner development towards the light, which wants to be nourished and supported. Reiki is a great, unconditional help and a source of power—a heavenly blessing.

Since I understand Reiki as a development process and not just as a technique, it is not my style to teach all three degrees in quick flow in a few weeks or even days. The time from the second to the third Reiki degree lasted up to 7 years for me personally, and only then was the time ripe for the next step, the inauguration to the Reiki Master. A minimum of one year of Reiki practice should, in my opinion, definitely pass between the second and third Reiki degrees.

The third Reiki degree is the full opening to the Reiki channel, and the initiation into the energy of the Master symbol is a big step in personal development. It is possible to make the third degree exclusively for your own Reiki practice and development and, thus, to have the full power of Reiki at your disposal. Others, on the other hand, train as re-masters in order to be able to give their own initiations in Reiki and seminars. In some traditions, this is referred to as a Reiki Master Teacher or as a fourth degree. In the third degree, further techniques for treatment are taught, including psycho-energetic surgery, as well as a particularly intensive breathing technique and meditation for the training of one's own energy body.

To be a Reiki master and to teach others in Reiki is a responsible task that we can only do justice to if we are willing to work on ourselves in accordance with the fourth Reiki rule of life, and this is certainly a wonderful development of one's own being towards the light. Daily meditation in the energy field of the Master symbol is one of many ways to promote development at all levels of one's being.

Building on the Master's degree, a whole series of other initiations are possible, sometimes referred to in the literature as the Reiki Grandmaster Degrees. This is another step on the path of Reiki, more to the higher Reiki Master degrees on the next page.

In the years 1999 to 2002, we learned that the founder of Reiki in Japan, Mikao Usui, also taught a system of mainly 3 Reiki degrees, but its content and objectives differ from the Western Reiki practice. The degrees and levels of Reiki, as originally taught by Usui Sensei himself in Japan, can be learned in the seminar URR & Usui Teate.

More Reiki Master Grades

With the big step to the Reiki Master Initiation, the road is far from over; on the contrary, now the learning really begins. All the more so when the Reiki

Master decides to teach others in Reiki and thus assumes a responsible task.

Building on the master's degree, other so-called Grandmaster grades have been developed by various people. So these are not symbols, and initiations that can be traced back to the founder of the Reiki, Mikao Usui, but rather further developments of Western Reiki masters, which are reflected in the inner level of spiritual and emotional development and can be very helpful with treatment.

I myself prefer to call these initiations "only" further or higher Reiki master degrees. Officially, at most, the president of the Usui Reiki Ryoho Gakkai would have the right to bear the title of Grand-Master. Some egos in the Reiki scene feel bigger with the Grand Master title, I deliberately do not want to promote this, so I call these initiations, as beautiful and powerful as they are, more master degrees.

The wisdom symbol comes from a Hessian Reiki master named Helmut Ernst and rightly bears his name. With our gaze into infinity, we are able to recognize higher connections and experience a serenity that alienates us from the consciousness of everyday life. For me, the first meditative practice with the wisdom symbol was as if the legacy of a thousand years of Buddhist meditation suddenly became available to me. The message of the wisdom symbol is: "the knowledge of this world is at your disposal." Wisdom, intuitive knowledge, spiritual guidance, and deep insight are promoted with this initiation and subsequent practice with the symbol.

The 4th Reiki degree (Radiance), the heart symbol, has the message "Light and love shine from my heart" and is beautiful for our heart. The energy of the symbol opens and purifies in the area of the heart and neck chakra and allows us to be back in love. The development of intellectual abilities is one side; one's own kindness of heart, and also the unconditional joy that comes with such a heart is certainly no less important. An injured or sorrowful heart can be led back into harmony and joy with the symbol of the heart. Another aspect is the ability to let heart energy radiate freely to the delight of others as well as of one's own.   According to my research, this symbol comes from the lineage of Barbara Weber-Ray, who made it from a source in Japan (Mieko Mitsui or Iris Ishikuro—who knows more exactly?) and integrated into their radiance system.

The 5th Reiki degree (Radiance), the neck chakra symbol, comes from the Barbara Ray line, i.e., from the A.I.R.A., later renamed Radiance. This Grand Master's Inauguration energizes, as the name suggests, the neck chakra. All areas and levels of expression, communication and truthfulness associated with this chakra are opened to the light. The message of this symbol is: "the divine powers are expressed." I find remarkable the connection between the opening of the neck chakra, the voice, and the quality of inner truthfulness. This can be experienced in the energy of this symbol and was also experienced by Ray's students (The Reiki Factor - Barbara Ray). As the phrase says so beautifully: "to be coherent."

The 5th Reiki degree, The Great Harmony, as well as the 6th degree, the Great Division, is attributed to two Reiki masters living in Germany; Raj Petter, and Jay Arjan Falk. There are many stories and rumors circulating about the origin of these degrees and unfortunately, there is no clear explanation of the origin of these degrees of Petter and Falk together. After repeated, extensive research also in the context of the emergence of these degrees from the years 1990 to 1992, the puzzle seems to me to be composed and the following about the origin of these two degrees crystallized:

The 5th and 6th degrees developed in two steps in their present form. A Buddhist monk named Serge Goldberg, a white-haired, nearly eighty-year-old American who had practiced Zen Buddhism for many decades, had the energies and mantras (or just self-initiation technique?) in the 1940s in a Japanese Reiki School. Raj Petter, who had been with Osho in India, met Serge Goldberg in India and brought these energies and mantras, as well as technology, to Europe from India.

In Germany, the energies and mantras were then passed on in a Reiki scene in the Frankfurt area in the early 1990s. A. Falk also came into contact with it and, according to Norbert Kuhl, simply took a Japanese dictionary and took symbols in Japanese kanji from it. Falk's own depiction varied, and his claim that the symbols were created in collaboration with a Japanese woman was unlikely because the sign of the mouth (a figure similar to the square) in the kanji would never be written in this way by any Japanese man in this form. So I suspect it was just a dictionary. With a ceremony, the symbols were then charged together with the mantras of Falk and the inauguration in the 5th and 6th degrees, as many Reiki masters have received since then, mainly in the German-speaking area, was created. This should have been 1993 or 94.

Anyway, the name of the 5th Grade, The Great Harmony, actually says it all — a beautiful healing harmony in the heart. Love is the greatest of all forces. Saint Amma of India says that 90% of all sufferings and illnesses are due to a lack of love, which is easy to understand. To be back in love with all my heart is healing on all levels par excellence. The great harmony is an energy, a force that makes the quality of heart and unity tangible. In treatments, I have been able to experience beautiful healings in people's hearts with this energy.

The 6th Reiki-Grade, The Great Division, is also from the line Serge Goldberg/ Petter & Falk and belongs together with the Great Harmony. Higher levels of awareness and clarity become tangible as soon as the essential is separated from the inessential.

The 7th and 8th Reiki degrees, are a further development of W. Keil and a Japanese student of mine; Dai Ji Yu, The Great Freedom, and Dai Hey Wa, The Great Peace. W. Wedge, initiated by Raj Petter in the Reiki Master, has received these two energies and with the help of Makiko, a Japanese Reiki student of mine, and a kanji dictionary, we have found matching symbols that are then found in a sacred ceremony of W. Keil and me (E bull) and that were connected to the energies. In the initiation ritual customary for all higher master degrees, since then, more precisely, since the year 2000, these initiations have been preserved in the 7th and 8th degrees. They have proved to be very blessed and particularly fine and high-swinging. They can be shared or passed on one after the other.

Dai Ji Yu, The Great Freedom, supports clarity in spirit, calm and free of attachment, and rejection to see things as they are. This is the freedom that lies in the sublime.

Dai Hey Wa, The Great Peace, gives security. Security in infinite, unconditional love. An "all-round feel-good," in its intensity far more powerful than what can be conveyed with the second or third Reiki degree. This is the power and divinity of the sublime, beyond all duality.

All initiations into the symbol of wisdom, as well as in the 4th, in both 5th, and in the 6th, 7th, and 8th degrees are an enrichment for any Reiki master both for his own inner development as well as for use in treatments. I am happy to pass on these degrees on a donation basis to interested Reiki masters, and appointments can be arranged individually. Prerequisite is an initiation in the 3rd Reiki degree, in the Reiki Master symbol Dai Ko Myo.

Often, a rather high price is demanded for these inaugurations, up to '40,000—for the heart chakra symbol at Barbara Weber-Ray. Giving these initiations on a donation basis, yes, that is still true for me, after I have initiated Reiki masters from many lines in it since about 1997. This is because I would like to make these degrees accessible to all interested parties, regardless of their material situation. What was not intended with the donation base, however, is that these grades will then be resold at double to almost five times the price of what was donated to me. From September 2003, the rule was, therefore, applied that the transmission of these initiations must not be more expensive than the donation made—which I actually take for granted, or don't?

All other Reiki master grades are very powerful and blessed, and they serve the spiritual nourishment and development of the master, e.g., in meditation. These particularly intense energies can also be used in treatments. It is an enrichment for every Reiki master with and without teaching skills. I am glad to be able to pass on this blessing.

And so I would like to conclude this text with a quote from Ayya Khema from her book with "Instructions of the Buddha to Happiness":

"What we do with love is well done. In reality, what we do with love is spiritually done. What we do without love can still look so spiritual, but has no spiritual content. Holiness is to be whole and nothing else. Bliss is bliss. We all have the skills to do so, but we have to work towards it and realize that it is possible... and leave this world a little more pure and beautiful than we found it."

CHAPTER 14

REIKI LIFE RULES

According to Buddhist tradition, the Reiki practice is started and ended with a prayer, a recitation. This prayer aligns one's own mind, clarifies the motivation for doing, and is thus an effective attunement and orientation in order to create a specific cause for a certain effect. Every Buddhist practice, such as a meditation on the medicine Buddha, begins with a prayer to clarify motivation. The text is always repeated at least three times, and the hands are folded in the prayer posture (Gassho) in front of the heart.

The full version of this text by Mikao Usui Sensei only became known in the West in the late 1990s. Ms. Hawayo Takata's previously learned version had been altered in the text. The Japanese version shown below was kindly provided by Ms. K. Koyama, former head of the Usui Reiki Ryoho Gakkai, in Tokyo.

Happiness, true well-being, healing at all levels is possible in the spirit of Reiki, in a spirit that has liberated itself to a universal being that clearly recognizes and lives in unity with the spiritual. In daily practice (especially today), certain guidelines such as peace, trust, gratitude, self-discipline and appreciation of others, hence the care of Buddhist (and also universally human) virtues in one's own thinking and feeling, are Prerequisite for attaining happiness. That is, to truly master his destiny, or, in the words of the New Age, to achieve self-realization. If the mind is in the right balance, the body must also follow and be healthy.

In my personal opinion, the Reiki rules of life contain typical Buddhist traits. So I would like to add a few suggestions from a Buddhist point of view.

At every moment (especially today — the clear alignment of attention to the here and now), we create our karma through thinking and acting on the inner and outer plane in the sense that it inevitably leaves traces in one's own consciousness. Sooner or later, we experience the effect of happiness or suffering. Therefore, at the beginning of an action, is a clarification of the orientation, the objective and the motivation. If we are aware that we are responsible for all the happiness and suffering we experience, a clear knowledge of what is to be promoted in one's own consciousness is most helpful. In this way, we can then promote happiness and reduce suffering. Qualities such as equanimity, trust, integrity and loving devotion to others are able to make our inner and outer lives healthier, more healing and lighter. Practice always takes place at this moment, in the here and now, and requires constant mindfulness, that is, work on ourselves.   Thus, the blessing of the Reiki practice can not only bring about a little relaxation, stress reduction, and relief of pain and illnesses, but also show a path that leads us into the light, to true happiness.

The Gyosei, poems of the Meiji Emperor, which, like the rules of life in Usui's Reiki practice, were quoted together, can be found here.

Another translation and interpretation of the Reiki rules of life, all of which originated in the original text of the Meiji Emperor, comes from the transmission line of the Reiki Jin-Kei-Do. This is perhaps the version that most corresponds to Buddhist thinking.

The Buddha taught that all life is painful, is Dukha (Being Unsatisfied). The existence of negative ominous emotions and thoughts in one's own mind as the cause of suffering is a fact that is to be recognized and transformed from this knowledge with clever methods. Thus compassion is the antidote to hatred, while doubt and worry are overcome by mindfulness in the here and now. In the end, we can free ourselves from all attachments, recognize our true being directly

115

and clearly, and thus free ourselves from many painful patterns. The practice of the art of life, to think and feel in a healing and happiness-bringing way, is what the Buddhist strives for at every moment, because in this way he can have a positive influence on his fate. Also noteworthy in this text is the reference to the direct connection between our thinking and feeling and our mental and physical health.

Dodrupchen teaches: "By practicing in this way, our spirit will become gentle. Our attitude will become tolerant. We will become very affable people. We will have a brave mindset. Our spiritual training will be free of obstacles. All adverse circumstances that occur will prove to be great and promise happiness. Our spirit will always be satisfied with the joy of inner peace. In order to practice the path of enlightenment in this age of decline, we must never be without the armor of this kind of training that transforms happiness and suffering into the path of enlightenment. If the suffering of worrying us does not plague us, then not only will other mental and emotional sufferings disappear - such as weapons that soldiers drop out of their hands - but in most cases, even the concrete negative forces, such as the physical diseases, disappear by themselves."

The saints of the past have said: "By not feeling anything and no one's dislike or dissatisfaction, our minds will remain untroubled. If our minds are not troubled, our energy will not be tarnished, and other elements of the body will not be bothered as well. Because of this inner calm and harmony, our minds will not be troubled, and the wheel of joy will continue to turn." They also said: "Just as it is easy for birds to inflict injuries on horses and donkeys with sore spots on their backs, negative forces will easily find an opportunity to harm those people whose beings are filled with fear of negative concern. But it will be hard to harm those whose beings are implemented by a strong positive attitude." (from Tulku Thondup, The Healing Power of the Spirit, Knaur Verlag, Men's Sana series. A book that explains health (well-being and happiness of life) from the point of view of a Tibetan Buddhist, and gives the reader many suggestions for a healing practice in everyday life. Not only suitable for Buddhists.)

The History Of Reiki

The story of Reiki, as a unique form of energy work, of healing with light, is inseparable from the person of its discoverer, a Japanese named Mikao Usui. And so I would like to begin the chapter on history with the life and work of this man to whom the world owes so much.

Mikao Usui was born on 15 May 1898. He was born in Yamagata District, Japan, in a Chiba clan Buddhist family with an ancient samurai tradition. Usui had a son and a daughter with his wife Sadako, née Suzuki. Professionally, he had experienced many things, he had worked in the civil service, and also as a businessman, reporter, secretary of a politician (bodyguard?), missionary and probation officer. As private secretary to the politician Shimpei Goto, Mikao Usui must have had good connections with the upper classes.

The time when Usui grew up in Japan was marked by renewal. After centuries of isolation, Japan reopened to foreign countries and to progress, but also to various ancient traditions that were not the former state religion of Shintoism. Belonged. A synthesis of old and new, this has also been the life path and life's work of Mikao Usui.

But he was not interested in worldly success, and perhaps he had been less interested in it. Mysticism and spirituality were of great importance to him, and he studied Kiko, the Japanese Qi Gong, to a high degree, interested in Chinese medicine, learned martial arts, among them Yagyu Shinkage Ryu

(Samurai Sword Fight) to the high degree of Menkyo Kaiden. He studied Tendai, Zen and Shingon Buddhism and also the ancient religion of Japan, Shinto. His interest was in medicine, psychology, fortune telling, and spiritual paths; he was an educated person with an awareness of inner qualities. He has also been to China and the West to learn, but it is quite possible that he has found much of his knowledge in the former imperial city of Kyoto with all its temples and libraries. Kyoto is a place with a very advanced cultural and spiritual heritage. Important companions of Mikao Usui include Morihei Ueshiba, the founder of Aikido martial arts, Onasiburo Deguchi, founder of the Oomoto religion, Toshihiro Eguchi, a good friend of Usui and also the founder of a religion, as well as Mokichi Okada, founder of the Oomoto religion. Johrei is the religion of spiritual light. Reiki is, therefore, a path of many that were created in this creative time in Japan.

CHAPTER 15

ON MOUNT KURAMA NEAR KYOTO

The life of Usui, for all his abilities and high education, was not particularly happy, and so he asked his spiritual teacher for advice, as is so common in Japanese culture. This led him to go on a retreat, i.e., to withdraw completely from the outer-worldly life and to practice "Shyu go," 21 days of fasting and meditation, a Buddhist practice that required a great deal of discipline and sincere effort. (The general form of meditation that Usui practiced is Zazen Shikan Taza, more on this in the URR and Usui Teate seminar.) A waterfall on Mount Kurama north of Kyoto was the perfect place to be undisturbed and practice. On the morning of the 21st day of this retreat, the light of Reiki unexpectedly came down to him and Reiki was born. Usui recognized and realized the Reiki healing method and had found himself, attaining a spiritual state of consciousness called "Anshin Ritsumei," which roughly means the following: one's own mind is perfectly at peace, it is clear what to do, nothing can disturb the inner peace and clarity anymore. I suspect this corresponds to Rigpa in Tibetan Buddhism.

This satori must have taken place between 1914 and 1922. The new healing method was first tested in the closest family circle, with such positive results, i.e., healing successes, that Usui decided to make this Ryoho, this healing method, freely accessible to all people. He deliberately did not want to hold them back as a sure source of income for his family and his descendants and kept them as a secret, thereby revealing his great spirit, his altruistic attitude to life. This is clear from the inscription (in German) at his grave in Tokyo.

In 1922, Usui had moved from Kyoto to Tokyo, and since Reiki had proved extremely helpful in various diseases and problems, he founded his first clinic, his first healing center. The interest in Reiki was immense, and people even had to queue in front of the house to get treatment from Usui or his co-workers. With his extraordinary abilities, Usui quickly became known throughout Japan, even though he explicitly did not want any publicity for Reiki. The treatments were open to all, which meant that they were not expensive if any fee was required.

In the few years that remained for his work with Reiki until his death, Usui taught and initiated well over 1000 people in this healing method, 17 of his students received the third grade, the 3rd or Shinpid degree.

The training in Reiki was initially divided into three degrees, and the first is called Shoden, the second Okuden and the third Shinpid. Shihan is the mystical teachings that are based on Shinpids. Only here, the disciple learned to give the initiations, Reiju. In addition, there are said to have been at least two higher master degrees, one without a name, the other meaning "bringing in the light." These empowerments can only be learned after many years of meditation practice and then passed on.

The second and even the third Reiki degree was awarded to the students only after a long-term collaboration with Usui Sensei, with their venerable teacher Usui. The student also had to demonstrate his sensitivity to being able to diagnose in the energy body (Byosen and Reiji Ho) in order to obtain further empowerment. The title "Sensei," venerable teacher, is bestowed on the teacher out of respect for his integrity and ability from the students.

Shoden, the first level of Reiki, was open to every student. People came to Usui to find healing; they received treatment from Usui and regular initiations (Reiju) in the first degree, in shodes. The higher degrees and empowerments, Okuden and Shinpids, and even more so, the even higher master degrees, were granted only after the student had demonstrated the necessary skills and character qualities. Years of cooperation and cooperation were a prerequisite, the Reiju, the attunement in Reiki, as well as a short form of Hatsurei Ho were regularly practiced. Even today, it may take up to ten years for a student in Usui Reiki Ryoho Gakkai to learn the second level, Okuden.

Mikao Usui placed great value on the spiritual side, the care of the inner spiritual qualities. His treatments were purely intuitive, sometimes he taught 5 head positions, as we have learned by now from the well over a 100-year-old student of Usui. He taught meditations and kotodamas, invocations to connect with special energies. If a student was not sensitive enough to do so, such as Hayashi, they were given the well-known 4 Reiki symbols as a tool.

Seventeen students have learned the Shinpid degree at Usui, 5 Buddhist nuns, 3 naval officers, and 9 other men, among them Eguchi, a close friend of Usui's. 50-70 students learned the first part (Zenki) of the 2nd degree, 30 also learned the 2nd part (Kouki) of Okuden.

Usui Sensei's goal was and is to improve the state of people's body, mind, and soul, and promote health, well-being and happiness. Reiki was, therefore, not only intended to cure illnesses and relieve pain but also to promote, in a holistic, spiritual sense, health at all levels of the human being and a healing mental state that means true happiness in life, and finally the enlightenment of obtaining liberation.

Shinto and Kiko were the basis for the energetic Reiki practice, and the Tendai Buddhism provided the spiritual background. It may be that Shingon and Zen also had influence, but only secondary. On this basis, Mikao Usui developed a very simple way of purifying and strengthening the human energy body and various forms of meditation, spiritual training. Usui taught a path to enlightenment and spiritual development, the pure laying on of hands, which has become so central in the West, was only a side issue. Weekly, the Reiju, the initiation in Reiki, was given. Religious texts and prayers were quoted together, it was about training one's own mind in mindfulness and pure presence and thus developing all hidden qualities beyond the ordinary.

The so-called Reiki Rules of Life, or Reiki ideals, which corresponded to the five principles of the Meiji Emperor, served as clear orientation for the Reiki practice. They were regularly recited at the beginning of the common practice. So did Gyosei, imperial poems for spiritual inspiration. Usui chose those Gyosei that were interesting and helpful as Kotodamas to lead the students into certain states. The Hikkei, the manual that Usui handed out to his students around 1920, contained the rules of life, gyosei, and meditations, but not hand positions.

Usui Reiki Ryoho Gakkai in Tokyo

Later, after Usui Sensei died of a brain stroke in 1926, the Usui Reiki Ryoho Gakkai, a society for the spread of the Reiki cure to Usui, was born in Tokyo. It has now been proven that Usui was not named as the first president of the Gakkai until after his death.

Mikao Usui himself is named as the first president of this Usui Reiki Ryoho Gakkai, and his successors were Juzaburo Ushida, Kan'ichi Taketomi, Houichi Wanami and Kimiko Koyama. The current President is Mr. Masaki Kondo. If anything, only Mr. Kondo could call himself the Grand Master or Head Teacher of Reiki, but such a term is unknown in Japan.

The teachings of the Gakkai, presented by Arjava Petter, William Rand, and Hiroshi Doi as the original Reiki of Mikao Usui, do not represent the practice as Usui Sensei himself taught it, but are a further development within the Gakkai.

The former president of the Gakkai in Tokyo, Mrs. Koyama, who is now also very well known to us, has the version of Usui Reiki Hikkei, a handbook that Usui partly gave to his students. The Usui Reiki Hikkei answers questions about Reiki, and an English translation can be found on Rick Rivard's website, "Reiki Threshold." The Hikkei also lists certain hand positions for a wide variety of diseases. According to the latest research in Japan (Usui Teate), the hand positions come from Hayashi's pen, hence the resemblance to the positions in his own Hikkei, and not at all from Usui himself. Students who learned directly from Usui—in contrast to the information of the Gakkai, which came from the 2nd hand and have been modified—have said that Usui taught only 5 special head positions, then the body was treated intuitively. More on the Usui Teate page.

The name Reiki consists of two kanjis, Japanese characters, Rei and Ki. There are several ways to interpret and translate these words:

Rei is the spiritual healing associated with spiritual growth.

Ki is the energy, the power to heal the mind and body. Here are the old and new definitions of the Kanjis:

A more literal translation, interpretation of the two Kanjis, is Rei: from heaven, the rain comes with life-giving energy, which is composed of three parts, light, love, and wisdom. Ki: on the earth, a shaman stands with his arms stretched out to heaven.

Reiki is, therefore, reception of light, love and wisdom from above, from heaven, and passing on to the people of the earth. This applies both to the initiation in Reiki and the treatment with Reiki.

Other sources - Kurama

Usui had certainly received inspiration from his studies of Zen Buddhism, as well as from Tendai and Shingon Buddhism. He knew other Japanese forms of light work and was probably also a member of the "Rei Jyutsu Ka," which was based at the foot of Mount Kurama. Usui Sensei was master (Menkyo Kaiden) in Japanese martial art called Yagyu Ryu. The account in some chapters of Usui's life story that he was secretary of a politician is probably a paraphrase of his work as a bodyguard.

Mount Kurama, an hour north of Kyoto, is a particularly sacred place in Japan, even called the spiritual heart of Japan. Many hundreds of temples are there, from all Japanese traditions, thus also their energies and helpers from the realm of light. Mountain Kurama is also a particularly sacred and blessed place for Japanese martial arts.

From 1922, Usui practiced Zen meditation for three years, several times he made a retreat, the frame of which is described in the Zazen Shikan Taza.

Perhaps the Satori that Usui experienced in March 1922 with the reception of Reiki on Mount Kurama was also inspired by the mystical history of the Kurama Sonten, which is connected to Mount Kurama and is still energetically effective there. The three deities of the Kurama Sonten embody different qualities and are represented by Sanskrit mantras. They are the divine attributes: light (Bishamon-Ten), love (Senju-Kannon), and power (Mao-Son). The mythology of the Kurama mountain has striking parallels to the degrees of Reiki! Sonten, depicted in kanji like the Reiki Master symbol, is the Universal Life Force, which permeates and nourishes the entire cosmos and manifests itself through the three properties of light, love and power.

The symbol of Senju-Kannon (a form of Avalokiteshvara, the thousand-armed Bodhisattva of consummate compassion) is the Hrih in Sanskrit and the source of the 2nd traditional Reiki symbol, the so-called mental symbol. It stands for the Amida Buddha (Amitabha), which is highly revered in Japan (Buddhism of the Pure Land). The Hrih embodies the blessing power of love in this trinity and is associated with the moon principle.

Bishamon-Ten is the power of light (light-strength is an essential property of the spirit of enlightenment) and is connected to the principle of the sun. Mao-Son is the third deity of the Kurama Sonata and means power. Mao-Son embodies the principle of the earth.

Also, the mantra of the master symbol is used daily in this temple on Mount Kurama for protection and invocation. The Dai Ko Myo, the Reiki Master symbol, represents the three principles of The Kurama Sonten: Love, Light and Power.

In 1923, Japan suffered a major, devastating earthquake, the Kanto earthquake, in which more than 100,000 people lost their lives. Mikao Usui was very committed to helping the victims to alleviate and heal their suffering with Reiki. To this end, he moved his clinic to the area of the earthquake in order to "extend the hands of love to the suffering people." This, too, shows that Usui Sensei was a man of the "Great Spirit" who, in a selfless manner, really practiced Bodhicitta, loving devotion. As an award for his services, Usui received a doctorate, honorably.

In 1926, Mikao Usui succumbed to a brain stroke. His grave is at the Saihoji Temple in Tokyo. Right next to the tomb is a stone with an inscription, soon also in the German translation of the inscription on the memorial stone, which reports on Usui's life and work. The discovery of this inscription, the discovery of Tokyo's Reiki-Gakkai, and two Japanese books on Reiki, made it possible at the end of the 20th century to obtain more coherent information about the history of Reiki and the life of its founder, Mikao Usui, in the West. The two Japanese Reiki books are the "Iyashi No Te" by Toshitaka Mochizuki and the "Iyashi No Gendai Reiki ho" by Hiroshi Doi. The book by Hiroshi Doi has been translated into English and is now available under the name "Modern Reiki Method for Healing." Further traditions of other Japanese Reiki teachers, who are not members of the Gakkai but can still be traced back to Mikao Usui or Chujiro Hayashi, have become known.

Thanksgivings/Proof of Source

Many have contributed to the news of the new information from Japan, most notably Frank Arjava Petter ("The Reiki Fire," "The Legacy of Dr.Usui" and "The Original Reiki Manual," all published by Windpferd- Verlag); and Hiroshi Doi, who trained with Usui Reiki Ryoho Gakkai now teaches this Reiki tradition in the West. I would also like to thank Andrew Bowling (Reiki History) from England for his history of Reiki and William Rand for Discovering the Roots of Reiki. At the end of 2000, the "Reiki

Compendium" of Lübeck, Petter, and Rand were published by Windpferd-Verlag on this topic. Another tradition of Buddhist Reiki practice is Buddho-Ener Sense. It is based on a line of Usui's student Hayashi.

Meanwhile, thanks to Chris Marsh and the insights about the Usui Teate, an even clearer picture of what Usui practiced and what he did not. In particular, I would like to thank Taggart King for his work and support.

Mikao Usui Sensei practiced daily the recitation of the Reiki rules of life and a short form of Hatsurei-Ho with his students and the initiation, which Reiju regularly repeats so that the ability to pass on Reiki has been increased more and more. It was clear to him that health and true happiness in life is inextricably linked to spiritual, inner values, and to spiritual development. He attached great importance to finding peace in one's own mind on the basis of ethically correct behavior and to act with a good heart and in inner silence as the great saints of all times for the good of men.

Reiki goes West, Hayashi & Takata

In this section, I would like to report a little about the transmission line from Reiki to the West. This line begins with Dr. Chujiro Hayashi and leads via Ms. Hawayo Takata to the U.S. and Europe.

Dr. Chujiro Hayashi, along with two other officers, Jusaburo Gyuda/Ushida and Ichi Taketomi, had been a student of Usui. Born in 1878, he had served as a commander in the Japanese Navy and as a doctor. In 1925, he learned (only) for 9 months Reiki from Mikao Usui and later ran a small Reiki clinic in Tokyo with 8 beds and 16 healers, who always gave two treatments. Hayashi had written his own manual, which was very similar in terms of treatment positions to Usui Reiki Hikkei. Both were probably made from Qi Gong materials, which were distributed in the Navy in 1927. The 3 officers were the founders of the Gakkai, but older students of Usui could not identify with what was practiced there. Eguchi was only with the Gakkai for 1 year, from which Hayashi probably learned the Reiju, the initiation, which he probably also modified.

The nationalist attitude of the "Officer Club" Reiki Ryoho Gakkai had even been too much for Hayashi, and so he went his own way and later was no longer a member of the Usui Reiki Ryoho Gakkai, but taught his own Reiki in the Hayashi Reiki Kenyu-kai from 1931. The spiritual dimension on which Usui Sensei had placed so much emphasis was not a central point for Hayashi, and he focused on the technique of laying on hands for the purpose of (physical) healing. Until his death in 1941, he had dedicated 17 students to the

Master's degree. One of his students was Ms. Hawayo Takata, who graduated from the Masters in 1938.

Hawayo Takata arrived on 24 May 1898. She was born in Hawaii, the daughter of Japanese immigrants. Life on the sugar cane plantation was hard and had made her sick. When Ms. Takata was in Tokyo in her mid-thirties for family reasons and was examined in a hospital, she was diagnosed with a tumor, gallstones, and appendicitis. She was already lying on the operating table when an inner voice told her impressively that surgery was not necessary. She asked the doctor for another possibility and learned about Hayashi's Reiki clinic, which was directly opposite the hospital. Instead of surgery, she received daily Reiki treatments, and was completely healed within 4 months. So convinced of Reiki, she wanted to learn it herself and was able to get Hayashi to give her the first degree in the spring of 1936. For a year, Hawayo Takata worked at the Reiki Clinic in Tokyo and received the second degree at the end.

In 1937 she returned to Hawaii and began her Reiki work there. In the winter of 1938, Hayashi inaugurated her master's degree. The political situation during the Second World War, when the US and Japan had been opponents of the war, may have been the reason that Ms. Takata made Mikao Usui a

Christian theologian. Pearl Harbour was all too well remembered by the Americans. In this situation, she would have had great difficulties if she had wanted to publicize something Japanese or Buddhist. So she began to tell a fairy tale and turned Usui into a Christian he definitely never was. The Reiki practice was also adapted for the West. The Hatsurei Ho, for example, she had learned from Hayashi but never passed it on to her students.

Usui would never have agreed that they, like other "line holders," would call themselves Reiki GrandMasters. He had deliberately created an open teaching system, called "Ronin," without leadership ambitions and open to anyone who had an interest.

Until her death in 1980, Hawayo Takata had inaugurated a total of 22 Reiki masters, including Barbara Ray, who founded the A.I.R.A., later Radiance, and her granddaughter Phyllis Lei Furumoto, who founded the Reiki Alliance. For a long time, these two organizations were leaders in the spread of Reiki in Europe, and it was only in the 1990s that it became possible to devote themselves as Free Reiki Masters to the mediation of Reiki. This abolished the high price level, one might also say, price cartels, and made Reiki accessible to an even greater number. The attempt by Phyllis Furumoto, the granddaughter of Ms. Takata, to patent the names "Reiki" and "Usui Reiki Shiki Ryoho" worldwide has fortunately failed because Reiki is now known and popular globally. The way in which she took on the role of Reiki GrandMaster is also doubtful.

Back to sources in Japan

At the beginning of the 21st century, a return to the origins of the Reiki takes place, and the western Reiki scene looks back at Japan to find out the true story about Reiki. In particular, it is thanks to William Rand, Arjava Petter, Rick Rivard and Hiroshi Doi that the so-called URR techniques have now become known in the West. Its source is the Gakkai, which—as we have seen—was created only after Usui's death and did not have the high spiritual level on which Usui had attached so much importance.

As at 2002, when I wrote these lines, 12 students of Usui still lived in Japan, the youngest of them was 107 years old. Chris Marsh has contact with them and passes on his research under the title "Usui Teate." I find this particularly exciting and I am very grateful that Taggart King has shared this teaching material with me in such a generous form, especially since Chris Marsh is very covered and has nothing to do with the Reiki boom. A move that makes him sympathetic to me and underlines his credibility.

Men Chhos Rei Kei, the medicine Dharma Reiki after Lama Yeshe alias R. Blackwell, another attempt to revive the original teaching of Usui, is based on documents found (allegedly?) in Japan. At the end of 2002, Lama Yeshe's details are questioned because he is not prepared to show the originals on which his teaching is based. It is now clear that Mr. Blackwell has proved to be implausible, as he has never kept all the promises to show the originals. Also, a high reincarnation, which he claims to be, is completely unknown in Bhutan and with H.H. Dalai Lama. Many of his students around the world have since distanced themselves from him, deleted the MDR websites and canceled the MDR seminars. The German Reiki Magazine, which had a translation of the book by Lama Yeshe alias R. Blackwell into German already in production, finally had to stop the project with financial losses.

Further development in the West

In addition to the attempts to go "back to the roots" to rediscover the original Reiki practice, there are also a number of developments in the West. The higher Reiki Master grades, also called "Grandmaster Degrees," are very beautiful energies.

And other styles, such as the Tibetan Reiki (William Lee Rand), Karuna Reiki, and Tera Mai Reiki (Kathleen

Milner), are also very interesting additions to the "traditional" western Reiki.

Many more Reiki styles could be mentioned, often interesting, and healing extensions. But some things in the esoteric scene should probably be called energy or light, not Reiki, because it has nothing to do with Reiki anymore. Partner merges and similar magic are not, in my opinion, a Reiki application. A very regrettable development through the publication of symbols and initiations in connection with a lack of respect and self-serving striving are distorted Forms of Reiki, which do not prove to be blessed. The term "Reiki" is not protected, and so, unfortunately, some things can run under the name Reiki, which do not deserve this name.

I hope that these excesses of the Reiki boom in the West are only very isolated cases, as Reiki is something so beautiful and blessed.

May the light prevail in order to make the world in which we all live a little more loving and peaceful. May we all strive for the great heritage of Usui to produce many salutary fruits in the spirit of its founder.

CPSIA information can be obtained
at www.ICGtesting.com
Printed in the USA
BVHW011407120722
641919BV00003BA/86

9 781801 446914